STAGE 3 KIDNEY DISEASE DIET COOKBOOK

The Ultimate Tasty Kidney-Friendly Recipes to Slow, Stop or Reverse Renal Disease

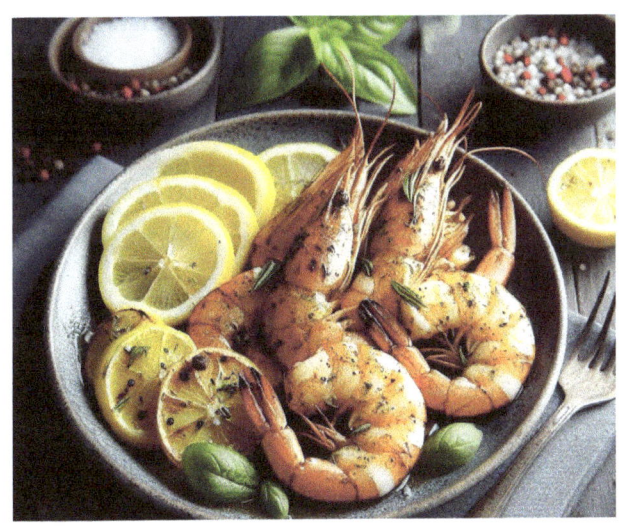

Deborah Weber

Copyright © Deborah Weber (2023)

The contents of this book are based on the author's research, knowledge, and experience. They are meant for educational purposes only and should not be taken as medical advice. Readers should consult their healthcare provider before making any changes to their health regimen.

Table of Contents

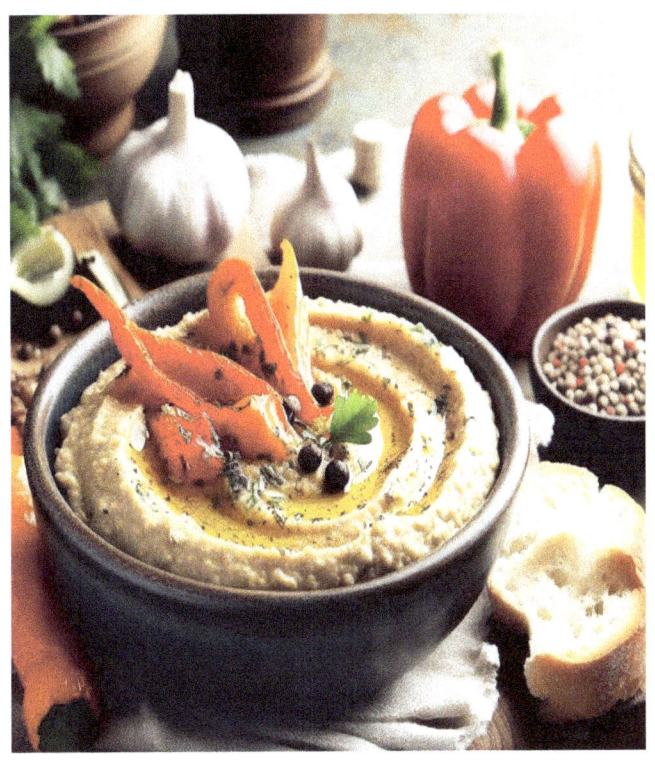

Introduction

When my Dad was diagnosed with Stage 3 kidney disease, our world shifted. It was as if life had suddenly whispered a secret that demanded our attention, urging us to embark on an uncharted journey of health and well-being. The doctor's words reverberated in our minds, leaving us with a mixture of uncertainty and determination. We were faced with a new reality, one that required not only medical treatment but also a profound transformation in our daily lives.

Amidst the plethora of doctor's appointments, lab results, and the swirling sea of medical information, there was a challenge that became both our concern and our mission: crafting a diet that aligned with my Dad's kidney health needs. It was a daunting endeavor, navigating the aisles of grocery stores, deciphering nutritional labels, and transforming familiar recipes into kidney-friendly wonders.

Yet, within this challenge lay an unexpected gift. The journey into the realm of kidney-conscious cuisine became a bond that tied us together, a shared adventure that forged a deeper connection between father and child. Together, we discovered the art of selecting nutrient-rich ingredients, the delight of experimenting with new flavors, and the joy of crafting meals that nourished not only the body but also the soul.

Through this journey, I learned that food is a language of love, a gesture that speaks volumes without uttering a word. Our kitchen became a place of creativity, a laboratory of healing, and a canvas of flavors waiting to be painted onto the plates.

As I reflect on those times, I realize that our experience isn't unique. Many families face similar challenges, grappling with how to best support their loved ones in their health journeys. This book is born from that shared experience. It's a compilation of recipes, meal plans, and insights that we wish we had when we first started down this road.

So, whether you're a patient, a caregiver, or simply someone seeking to embrace a kidney-friendly lifestyle, I invite you to join me on this journey. Let these pages be your guide, your inspiration, and your ally in crafting meals that not only nurture the body but also honor the soul. Let's embark together on a culinary adventure that bridges the gap between health and indulgence, and let's savor every step of the way.

Chapter 1: Understanding and Managing Stage 3 Kidney Disease

Welcome to the illuminating exploration of stage 3 kidney disease, a critical juncture in the journey of kidney health. In this section, we embark on a detailed journey to unravel the complexities of this condition. Armed with knowledge, you'll be better equipped to comprehend its nuances, implications, and the path forward.

The Significance of Stage 3

Stage 3 kidney disease is a pivotal phase in the spectrum of kidney dysfunction. It signifies a moderate decline in kidney function and warrants thorough understanding due to its potential impact on overall health. At this juncture, your kidneys are tasked with filtering waste and excess fluids less effectively, potentially leading to the accumulation of harmful substances in your body.

The Role of Glomerular Filtration Rate (GFR)

A key marker in assessing kidney health is the Glomerular Filtration Rate (GFR). This rate measures how efficiently your kidneys are filtering waste from your blood. Stage 3 kidney disease is characterized by a GFR of 30-59 ml/min, indicating a notable decrease in kidney function. GFR serves as a crucial indicator of the progression and severity of kidney dysfunction.

Progressive Nature of Kidney Disease

Understanding the progressive nature of kidney disease is pivotal. Stage 3 represents a transition from the early stages of kidney dysfunction, such as stage 1 and 2, to a more advanced phase. The pace of progression can vary from person to person, making it imperative to address the condition proactively.

Causes

Stage 3 kidney disease is often the result of a culmination of factors that impact kidney function over time. Some of the primary causes include:

- **High Blood Pressure (Hypertension)**: Uncontrolled high blood pressure places excessive strain on the blood vessels in the kidneys, impairing their ability to filter blood effectively. Over time, this can lead to kidney damage and reduced function.

- **Diabetes**: Diabetes is a significant contributor to kidney disease. Elevated blood sugar levels can damage the small blood vessels and filtering units (glomeruli) of the kidneys, resulting in reduced kidney function.

- **Kidney Infections and Inflammation**: Infections, such as urinary tract infections, can spread to the kidneys and cause inflammation. Chronic inflammation is known to lead to scarring and impaired kidney function.

- **Glomerulonephritis**: This term refers to inflammation of the kidney's filtering units (glomeruli). It can be caused by infections, immune system disorders, and other factors, eventually leading to kidney damage.

- **Polycystic Kidney Disease (PKD)**: A genetic disorder characterized by the growth of fluid-filled cysts in the kidneys, PKD can progressively impair kidney function.

- **Kidney Stones**: Recurrent kidney stones can cause damage to the kidney tissue and impair its function if left untreated.

Risk Factors

Certain factors increase the likelihood of developing stage 3 kidney disease. Recognizing these risk factors can guide preventive measures and early intervention:

- **Age**: Kidney function naturally declines with age, making older individuals more susceptible to kidney disease.

- **Family History**: A family history of kidney disease or related conditions increases the risk of developing kidney problems.

- **Gender**: Men are generally at a higher risk for kidney disease compared to women.

- **Ethnicity**: Some ethnic groups, such as African Americans, Hispanics, and Native Americans, are at an increased risk of kidney disease.

- **High Blood Pressure and Diabetes**: Individuals with uncontrolled high blood pressure and diabetes are at a significantly higher risk of developing kidney disease.

- **Obesity**: Excess weight strains various organs, including the kidneys, potentially leading to reduced kidney function.

- **Smoking**: Smoking damages blood vessels and increases the risk of kidney disease, particularly in individuals with pre-existing conditions.

- **Cardiovascular Disease**: Heart-related conditions can impact kidney health due to shared risk factors and circulatory connections.

- **Exposure to Certain Medications and Toxins**: Prolonged use of certain medications, as well as exposure to environmental toxins, can harm kidney function.

Recognizing the Symptoms

Stage 3 kidney disease often presents a range of symptoms that might not be immediately evident. The subtlety of these symptoms underscores the importance of regular health check-ups and open communication with healthcare professionals. While symptoms can vary from person to person, some common indicators include:

1. Fatigue and Weakness:
Feeling consistently fatigued or weak is a frequent complaint among individuals with stage 3 kidney disease. The build-up of waste products in the body due to impaired kidney function can contribute to this overwhelming sense of tiredness.

2. Fluid Retention and Swelling (Edema):
As kidney function declines, the body's ability to eliminate excess fluids becomes compromised. This can result in swelling, especially in the legs, ankles, and feet. Edema is often more noticeable in the later stages of stage 3 kidney disease.

3. Changes in Urination:
Alterations in urination patterns are often indicative of kidney dysfunction. You may experience changes such as increased or decreased urine output, foamy urine, or frequent nighttime urination.

4. Unexplained Weight Loss:

Weight loss unrelated to changes in diet or activity level can be a sign of kidney disease. The body's ability to eliminate waste products is compromised, leading to unintended weight loss.

5. Changes in Appetite and Taste:

A decrease in appetite or a metallic taste in the mouth can occur due to the accumulation of waste products in the bloodstream. This can affect your sense of taste and overall appetite.

6. Anemia:

Kidney disease can lead to a decrease in the production of red blood cells, resulting in anemia. Anemia may manifest as fatigue, pale skin, shortness of breath, and dizziness.

7. Bone Health Issues:

Impaired kidney function affects the body's ability to convert vitamin D into its active form, which can lead to bone health issues, such as bone pain and an increased risk of fractures.

8. High Blood Pressure:

Kidneys play a vital role in regulating blood pressure. As kidney function declines, blood pressure can increase, contributing to cardiovascular complications.

9. Cognitive Changes:
In some cases, cognitive changes such as difficulty concentrating, memory problems, and confusion can arise due to waste accumulation affecting brain function.

Navigating Nutritional Guidelines

Balancing Nutritional Needs:

Nutrition is a cornerstone in managing stage 3 kidney disease. Proper dietary choices can help alleviate symptoms, slow disease progression, and minimize the risk of complications. The following guidelines can serve as a blueprint for creating a kidney-friendly diet plan:

1. Controlled Protein Intake:
Protein is essential for growth and repair, but excessive protein intake can strain compromised kidneys. Opt for high-quality protein sources like lean meats, poultry, fish, eggs, and plant-based options such as legumes, tofu, and quinoa. Monitor your protein intake to avoid overburdening your kidneys.

2. Sodium Management:
Reducing sodium intake helps control blood pressure and minimize fluid retention. Reduced intake of processed foods, canned soups, and salty

snacks, is equally important. Opt for fresh, whole foods and use herbs and spices to enhance flavor without excessive salt.

3. Phosphorus Regulation:
Phosphorus balance is vital for kidney health. Limit high-phosphorus foods such as dairy products, nuts, seeds, and processed foods with phosphorus additives. Opt for low-phosphorus alternatives and consume dairy in moderation.

4. Potassium Moderation:
Balancing potassium levels helps prevent heart and muscle complications. Limit high-potassium foods like bananas, oranges, tomatoes, and potatoes. Choose lower-potassium fruits and vegetables and follow portion guidelines.

5. Fluid Control:
Individual fluid needs vary, but excess fluid intake can strain weakened kidneys. Consult with your healthcare provider to determine your specific fluid allowance based on your kidney function and overall health.

6. Healthy Fats:
Incorporate heart-healthy fats like olive oil, avocados, nuts, and seeds. These fats support overall health without overburdening the kidneys.

7. Others

Other important nutritional guidelines include monitoring vitamins and minerals, controlling portion sizes to prevent overloading your kidneys, and regularly monitoring kidney function through blood tests and staying in touch with your healthcare team is crucial.

Chapter 2: Breakfast Recipes

Creamy Oatmeal with Fresh Berries
Mediterranean Chickpea Salad
Spinach and Mushroom Frittata
Greek Yogurt Parfait with Mixed Berries
Mixed Berry Smoothie
Berry Chia Pudding
Caprese Salad
Zucchini Noodles with Pesto
Apple Walnut Salad with Yogurt Dressing
Cucumber and Tomato Salad

Creamy Oatmeal with Fresh Berries

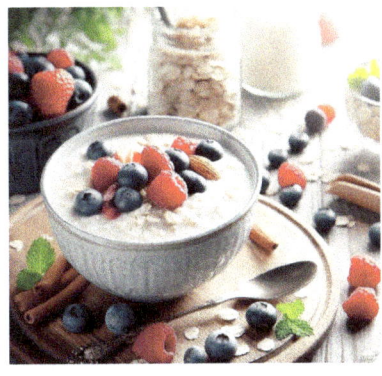

Preparation Time: 5 Minutes
Cooking Time: 10 minutes
Portion Size: 1 bowl

Ingredients:
- 1/2 cup rolled oats
- 1 cup water
- 1/2 cup low-fat milk
- 1/4 teaspoon cinnamon
- 1/2 cup mixed fresh berries (blueberries, strawberries, raspberries)
- 1 tablespoon chopped nuts (almonds, walnuts)

Instructions:
1. In a saucepan, bring water to a boil, and then add rolled oats, reducing heat to simmer.

2. Cook oats for about 5 minutes, stirring occasionally until creamy and thick.
3. Stir in low-fat milk and cinnamon, and cook for an additional 2 minutes.
4. Remove the mixture from heat and let it sit for a minute.
5. Top with mixed fresh berries and chopped nuts before serving.

Nutritional Value (Approximate per serving):
Calories: 250
Total Fat: 5g
Saturated Fat: 1g
Cholesterol: 5mg
Sodium: 100mg
Total Carbohydrates: 45g
Dietary Fiber: 6g
Sugars: 10g
Protein: 8g

Mediterranean Chickpea Salad

Preparation Time: 10 Minutes
Cooking Time: 0 minutes (no cooking required)
Portion Size: 1 bowl

Ingredients:
- 1 can (15 oz) of chickpeas (should be drained and rinsed)
- 1/2 cucumber, diced
- 1/2 red bell pepper, diced
- 1/4 red onion, finely chopped
- 1/4 cup crumbled feta cheese
- 2 tablespoons chopped fresh parsley
- Juice of 1 lemon
- 2 tablespoons olive oil
- Salt and pepper to taste

Instructions:
1. In a bowl, combine chickpeas, diced cucumber, red bell pepper, red onion, crumbled feta cheese, and chopped parsley.
2. Lemon juice, olive oil, salt, and pepper are whisked together in a small bowl.
3. The dressing should be drizzled over the salad and toss to combine.

Nutritional Value (Approximate per serving):
Calories: 200
Total Fat: 7g
Saturated Fat: 1g
Cholesterol: 0mg
Sodium: 350mg
Total Carbohydrates: 28g
Dietary Fiber: 9g
Sugars: 5g
Protein: 8g

Spinach and Mushroom Frittata

Preparation Time: 10 Minutes
Cooking Time: 20 minutes
Portion Size: 1 slice

Ingredients:
- 4 large eggs
- 1 cup fresh spinach, chopped
- 1/2 cup mushrooms, sliced
- 1/4 cup low-fat shredded cheese
- 1/4 teaspoon black pepper
- 1/4 teaspoon garlic powder

Instructions:
1. Preheat the oven to 350°F (175°C).
2. In a bowl, whisk together eggs, black pepper, and garlic powder.
3. In a non-stick skillet, sauté mushrooms until they release their moisture.
4. Add chopped spinach and cook until wilted.
5. Pour the egg mixture over the veggies and cook on low for 2-3 minutes.
6. Sprinkle shredded cheese on top and transfer the skillet to the preheated oven.

7. Bake for about 10-12 minutes or until the frittata is set in the center.

Nutritional Value (Approximate per serving):
Calories: 150
Total Fat: 10g
Saturated Fat: 4g
Cholesterol: 200mg
Sodium: 350mg
Total Carbohydrates: 6g
Dietary Fiber: 2g
Sugars: 2g
Protein: 10g

Greek Yogurt Parfait with Mixed Berries

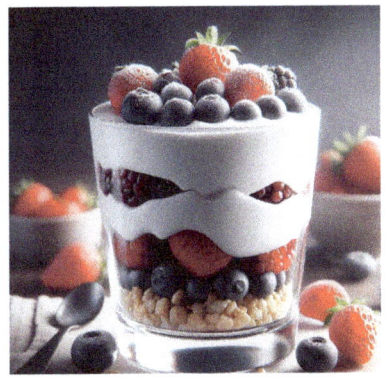

Preparation Time: 5 Minutes
Cooking Time: 0 minutes (no cooking required)
Portion Size: 1 parfait

Ingredients:

- 1 cup plain Greek yogurt
- 1/2 cup mixed berries (blueberries, strawberries, raspberries)
- 2 tablespoons chopped nuts (almonds, walnuts)
- 1 tablespoon honey (optional)

Instructions:

1. Greek yogurt, mixed berries, and chopped nuts are layered in a bowl or glass.
2. Honey is then drizzled on top for added sweetness if it is so desired.
3. Enjoy as a wholesome breakfast or snack.

Nutritional Value (Approximate per serving):
Calories: 200
Total Fat: 5g
Saturated Fat: 1g
Cholesterol: 10mg
Sodium: 100mg
Total Carbohydrates: 30g
Dietary Fiber: 4g
Sugars: 20g
Protein: 10g

Mixed Berry Smoothie

Preparation Time: 5 Minutes
Cooking Time: 0 minutes (no cooking required)
Portion Size: 1 smoothie

Ingredients:
- 1/2 cup mixed berries (blueberries, strawberries, raspberries)
- 1/2 banana
- 1/2 cup plain Greek yogurt
- 1/2 cup of low-fat milk or dairy-free alternative
- 1 tablespoon honey
- 1/2 teaspoon vanilla extract

Instructions:
1. Place mixed berries, banana, Greek yogurt, milk, honey, and vanilla extract in a blender.
2. Blend until smooth and creamy.
3. Pour into a glass and enjoy as a nutritious snack or breakfast option.

Nutritional Value (Approximate per serving):
Calories: 180
Total Fat: 2g
Saturated Fat: 0g
Cholesterol: 5mg
Sodium: 100mg
Total Carbohydrates: 40g
Dietary Fiber: 8g
Sugars: 24g
Protein: 6g

Berry Chia Pudding

Preparation Time: 10 Minutes
Cooking Time: 0 minutes (refrigeration required)
Portion Size: 1 serving

Ingredients:
- 1/4 cup chia seeds
- 1 cup of low-fat milk or any other dairy-free alternative
- 1/2 cup mixed berries (blueberries, strawberries, raspberries)
- 1 tablespoon honey
- 1/2 teaspoon vanilla extract

Instructions:
1. In a bowl, mix milk and chia seeds. Then stir well and let it sit for 5 minutes.
2. Stir the mixture again to prevent clumping.
3. The mixture is covered and refrigerated overnight or for at least 4 hours.
4. In the morning, top the chia pudding with mixed berries, drizzle with honey, and sprinkle with vanilla extract.

Nutritional Value (Approximate per serving):
Calories: 200
Total Fat: 8g
Saturated Fat: 2g
Cholesterol: 0mg
Sodium: 50mg
Total Carbohydrates: 25g
Dietary Fiber: 8g
Sugars: 12g
Protein: 6g

Caprese Salad

Preparation Time: 10 Minutes
Cooking Time: 0 minutes (no cooking required)
Portion Size: 1 serving

Ingredients:
- 2 large tomatoes, sliced
- 1 cup fresh mozzarella cheese, sliced
- 1/4 cup fresh basil leaves
- 2 tablespoons balsamic glaze
- 1 tablespoon extra-virgin olive oil
- Salt and pepper to taste

Instructions:
1. Arrange tomato slices and mozzarella cheese slices on a serving platter.
2. Fresh basil leaves are tucked between the tomato and cheese slices.
3. Balsamic glaze and extra-virgin olive oil are drizzled over the salad.
4. Season with salt and pepper before serving.

Nutritional Value (Approximate per serving):
Calories: 250
Total Fat: 20g
Saturated Fat: 7g
Cholesterol: 30mg
Sodium: 300mg
Total Carbohydrates: 8g
Dietary Fiber: 2g
Sugars: 4g
Protein: 10g

Zucchini Noodles with Pesto

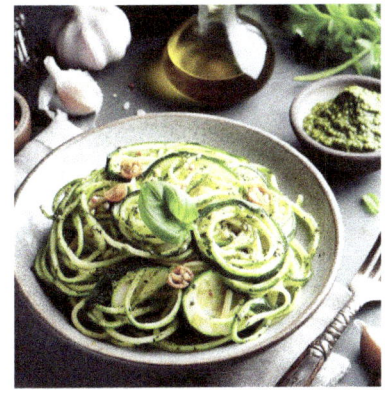

Preparation Time: 15 Minutes
Cooking Time: 10 minutes
Portion Size: 1 serving

Ingredients:

- 2 medium zucchinis, spiralized into noodles
- 1/4 cup prepared pesto sauce
- 1/4 cup cherry tomatoes, halved
- 2 tablespoons grated Parmesan cheese
- 1 tablespoon chopped fresh basil
- Salt and pepper to taste

Instructions:

1. In a skillet, sauté zucchini noodles for 1-2 minutes until slightly softened.
2. Add prepared pesto sauce and cherry tomato halves, and toss to coat.

3. The mixture is cooked for an additional 1-2 minutes until heated through.
4. Remove from heat and sprinkle with grated Parmesan cheese and chopped fresh basil.

Nutritional Value (Approximate per serving):
Calories: 250
Total Fat: 20g
Saturated Fat: 3g
Cholesterol: 5mg
Sodium: 300mg
Total Carbohydrates: 10g
Dietary Fiber: 3g
Sugars: 5g
Protein: 8g

Apple Walnut Salad with Yogurt Dressing

Preparation Time: 10 Minutes
Cooking Time: 0 minutes (no cooking required)
Portion Size: 1 salad

Ingredients:
- 2 cups mixed salad greens
- 1 apple, sliced
- 1/4 cup chopped walnuts
- 1/4 cup dried cranberries
- 1/4 cup crumbled goat cheese (optional)

For the Yogurt Dressing:
- 1/4 cup plain Greek yogurt
- 1 tablespoon apple cider vinegar
- 1 tablespoon honey
- Salt and pepper to taste

Instructions:
1. In a large bowl, combine mixed salad greens, sliced apple, chopped walnuts, dried cranberries, and crumbled goat cheese.

2. In a separate small bowl, whisk together Greek yogurt, apple cider vinegar, honey, salt, and pepper.
3. The yogurt dressing is drizzled over the salad and tossed to coat.

Nutritional Value (Approximate per serving):
Calories: 220
Total Fat: 12g
Saturated Fat: 2g
Cholesterol: 5mg
Sodium: 150mg
Total Carbohydrates: 25g
Dietary Fiber: 5g
Sugars: 18g
Protein: 6g

Cucumber and Tomato Salad

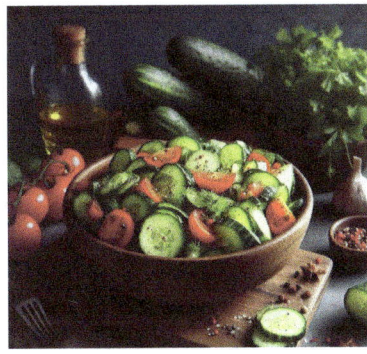

Preparation Time: 10 Minutes
Cooking Time: 0 minutes (no cooking required)
Portion Size: 1 serving

Ingredients:
- 1 cucumber, diced
- 1 cup cherry tomatoes, halved
- 1/4 red onion, thinly sliced
- 2 tablespoons chopped fresh dill
- 2 tablespoons olive oil
- 1 tablespoon red wine vinegar
- Salt and pepper to taste

Instructions:
1. In a bowl, combine diced cucumber, cherry tomatoes, red onion, and chopped dill.
2. In a small bowl, whisk together red wine vinegar, olive oil, salt, and pepper.

3. Toss the dressing with the salad ingredients and let it marinate for a few minutes before serving.

Nutritional Value (Approximate per serving):
Calories: 60
Total Fat: 3g
Saturated Fat: 0g
Cholesterol: 0mg
Sodium: 100mg
Total Carbohydrates: 8g
Dietary Fiber: 2g
Sugars: 4g
Protein: 2g

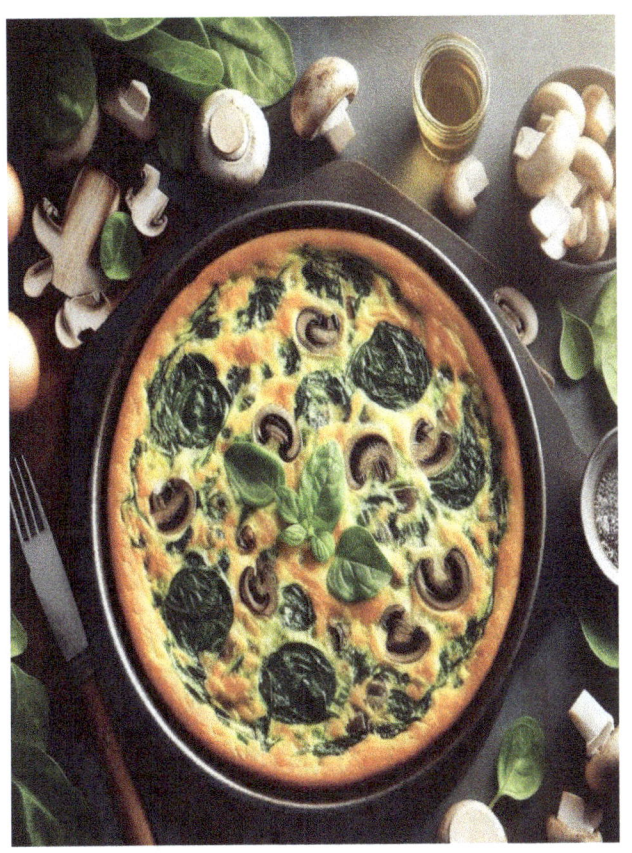

Chapter 3: Lunch Recipes

Grilled Chicken Salad with Lemon Vinaigrette
Lentil and Vegetable Soup
Black Bean and Corn Salad
Turkey and Vegetable Skewers
Roasted Beet and Goat Cheese Salad
Italian Bean Salad
Mushroom and Spinach Stuffed Chicken Breast
Quinoa Stuffed Bell Peppers
Baked Salmon with Herbed Quinoa
Lemon Herb Grilled Shrimp

Grilled Chicken Salad with Lemon Vinaigrette

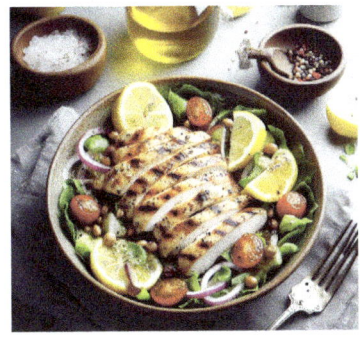

Preparation Time: 15 Minutes
Cooking Time: 15 minutes
Portion Size: 1 Salad

Ingredients:

- 4 oz boneless, skinless chicken breast
- 2 cups mixed salad greens
- 1/4 cup cherry tomatoes, halved
- 1/4 cucumber, sliced
- 1/4 red onion, thinly sliced
- 1 tablespoon chopped fresh herbs (parsley, basil)

Instructions:

1. The grill or grill pan is preheated over medium-high heat.
2. Season chicken breast with a pinch of salt and pepper.

3. Grill chicken for about 6-7 minutes per side or until fully cooked.
4. Let chicken rest for a few minutes, then slice it into thin strips.
5. Mixed salad greens, cherry tomatoes, cucumber, and red onion are then combined in a bowl.
6. Top with sliced grilled chicken and chopped fresh herbs.
7. Drizzle with lemon vinaigrette before serving.

Nutritional Value (Approximate per serving):
Calories: 350
Total Fat: 18g
Saturated Fat: 3g
Cholesterol: 85mg
Sodium: 400mg
Total Carbohydrates: 15g
Dietary Fiber: 4g
Sugars: 5g
Protein: 32g

Lentil and Vegetable Soup

Preparation Time: 15 Minutes
Cooking Time: 30 minutes
Portion Size: 1 bowl

Ingredients:
- **Preheat 1 cup of dried green lentils (must be well rinsed and drained)**
- **4 cups low-sodium vegetable broth**
- **1 carrot, diced**
- **1 celery stalk, diced**
- **1/2 onion, chopped**
- **2 cloves garlic, minced**
- **1 teaspoon dried thyme**
- **Salt and pepper to taste**

Instructions:
1. In a large pot, sauté onion, carrot, and celery until slightly softened.
2. Minced garlic is added to the mixture and cooked for another minute.
3. Add lentils, vegetable broth, and dried thyme.
4. The mixture is brought to a boil, the heat reduced, and the mixture is allowed to

simmer for about 20-25 minutes or until the lentils are tender.

5. Season with salt and pepper before serving.

Nutritional Value (Approximate per serving):
Calories: 180
Total Fat: 2g
Saturated Fat: 0.3g
Cholesterol: 0mg
Sodium: 350mg
Total Carbohydrates: 32g
Dietary Fiber: 12g
Sugars: 6g
Protein: 10g

Black Bean and Corn Salad

Preparation Time: 10 Minutes
Cooking Time: 0 minutes (no cooking required)
Portion Size: 1 cup

Ingredients:
- 1 can (15 oz) of black beans (drained and rinsed)
- 1 cup of corn kernels (any of fresh, frozen, or canned can be used)
- 1/2 red bell pepper, diced
- 1/4 red onion, finely chopped
- 1/4 cup chopped fresh cilantro
- Juice of 1 lime
- 1 tablespoon olive oil
- Salt and pepper to taste

Instructions:
1. In a bowl, combine black beans, corn, red bell pepper, red onion, and chopped cilantro.
2. Olive oil, lime juice, salt, and pepper, are all whisked together in a separate small bowl.
3. Pour the dressing over the salad and then toss it to combine.

4. The flavors are allowed to meld for about 15 minutes before serving.

Turkey and Vegetable Skewers

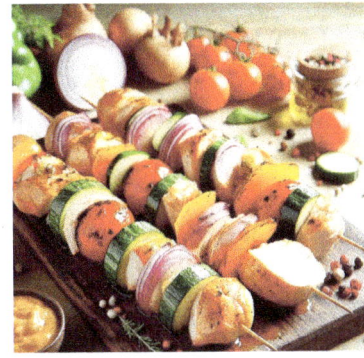

Preparation Time: 10 Minutes
Cooking Time: 20 minutes
Portion Size: 1 cup

Ingredients:

- 8 oz lean ground turkey
- 1/2 zucchini, sliced
- 1/2 red onion, cut into chunks
- 1/2 bell pepper (any color), cut into chunks
- 1 tablespoon olive oil
- 1 teaspoon of dried Italian herbs (any of oregano, basil, thyme will do)
- Salt and pepper to taste

Instructions:

1. The grill or grill pan is preheated over medium-high heat.
2. In a bowl, mix ground turkey with dried Italian herbs, salt, and pepper.

46

3. Shape the turkey mixture into small meatballs.
4. Thread the turkey meatballs, zucchini slices, red onion, and bell pepper onto skewers.
5. Brush skewers with olive oil and grill for about 10-12 minutes, turning occasionally, until turkey is cooked through.

Nutritional Value (Approximate per serving):
Calories: 60
Total Fat: 3g
Saturated Fat: 0.5g
Cholesterol: 0mg
Sodium: 200mg
Total Carbohydrates: 8g
Dietary Fiber: 3g
Sugars: 2g
Protein: 3g

Roasted Beet and Goat Cheese Salad

Preparation Time: 15 Minutes
Cooking Time: 1 hour (for roasting beets)
Portion Size: 1 salad

Ingredients:

- 2 medium beets, peeled and diced
- 4 cups mixed salad greens
- 1/4 cup crumbled goat cheese
- 2 tablespoons chopped walnuts
- 2 tablespoons balsamic vinegar
- 1 tablespoon olive oil
- 1 teaspoon honey
- Salt and pepper to taste

Instructions:

1. Preheat the oven to 400°F (200°C).
2. Toss diced beets with olive oil, salt, and pepper.
3. Spread beets on a baking sheet and roast for about 20-25 minutes or until tender.
4. In a bowl, combine mixed salad greens, roasted beets, crumbled goat cheese, and chopped walnuts.

5. In a small bowl, whisk together olive oil, honey, balsamic vinegar, olive oil, salt, and pepper. Drizzle over the salad before serving.

Nutritional Value (Approximate per serving):
Calories: 200
Total Fat: 12g
Saturated Fat: 5g
Cholesterol: 20mg
Sodium: 300mg
Total Carbohydrates: 20g
Dietary Fiber: 5g
Sugars: 12g
Protein: 6g

Italian Bean Salad

Preparation Time: 15 Minutes
Cooking Time: 0 minutes (no cooking required)
Portion Size: 1 cup

Ingredients:
- 1 can (15 oz) of low-sodium kidney beans, drained and rinsed
- 1 can (15 oz) low-sodium cannellini beans (drained and rinsed)
- 1/2 cup diced red onion
- 1/2 cup diced bell pepper (any color)
- 1/4 cup chopped fresh parsley
- 2 tablespoons olive oil
- 2 tablespoons red wine vinegar
- 1 teaspoon dried Italian herbs (any of oregano, basil or thyme)
- Salt and pepper to taste

Instructions:
1. In a large bowl, combine kidney beans, cannellini beans, diced red onion, diced bell pepper, and chopped parsley.

2. In a small bowl, whisk together olive oil, red wine vinegar, dried Italian herbs, salt, and pepper.
3. Toss the dressing with the bean mixture and let it marinate for a few minutes before serving.

Nutritional Value (Approximate per serving):
Calories: 180
Total Fat: 6g
Saturated Fat: 1g
Cholesterol: 0mg
Sodium: 350mg
Total Carbohydrates: 25g
Dietary Fiber: 7g
Sugars: 4g
Protein: 7g

Mushroom and Spinach Stuffed Chicken Breast

Preparation Time: 20 Minutes
Cooking Time: 30 minutes
Portion Size: 1 stuffed chicken breast

Ingredients:

- 2 boneless, skinless chicken breasts
- 1 cup baby spinach leaves
- 1/2 cup sliced mushrooms
- 1/4 cup low-fat mozzarella cheese
- 1/4 teaspoon garlic powder
- Salt and pepper to taste

Instructions:

1. Preheat the oven to 375°F (190°C).
2. A horizontal slit is made in each chicken breast to create a pocket.
3. Fill each pocket with baby spinach, sliced mushrooms, and mozzarella cheese.
4. Season the chicken breasts with garlic powder, salt, and pepper.
5. Place the stuffed chicken breasts on a baking sheet and bake for about 25-30 minutes or until cooked through.

Nutritional Value (Approximate per serving):
Calories: 350
Total Fat: 15g
Saturated Fat: 6g
Cholesterol: 100mg
Sodium: 450mg
Total Carbohydrates: 10g
Dietary Fiber: 2g
Sugars: 4g
Protein: 40g

Quinoa Stuffed Bell Peppers

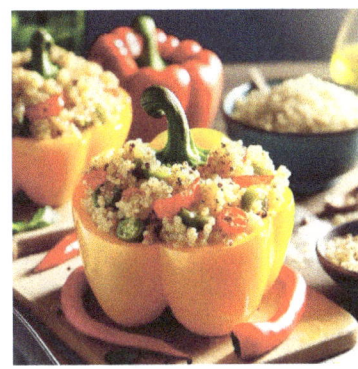

Preparation Time: 20 Minutes
Cooking Time: 40 minutes
Portion Size: 1 stuffed pepper

Ingredients:

- 2 large bell peppers, (they should both be halved and their seeds removed)
- 1 cup cooked quinoa
- 1/2 cup of canned low-sodium black beans, (they should be rinsed and drained)
- 1/2 cup diced tomatoes
- 1/4 cup diced red onion
- 1/4 cup chopped fresh parsley
- 1 teaspoon ground cumin
- 1/2 teaspoon chili powder
- 1/4 cup low-fat shredded cheese (optional)

Instructions:

1. Preheat the oven to 375°F (190°C).

2. In a bowl, combine cooked quinoa, black beans, diced tomatoes, red onion, parsley, ground cumin, and chili powder.
3. Fill the bell pepper halves with the quinoa mixture and place them in a baking dish.
4. Shredded cheese can be sprinkled on top of each stuffed pepper if so desired.
5. The stuffed peppers are then baked for about 20-25 minutes or until they are tender and the filling is heated through.

Nutritional Value (Approximate per serving):
Calories: 250
Total Fat: 6g
Saturated Fat: 1g
Cholesterol: 0mg
Sodium: 400mg
Total Carbohydrates: 42g
Dietary Fiber: 8g
Sugars: 8g
Protein: 9g

Baked Salmon with Herbed Quinoa

Preparation Time: 15 Minutes
Cooking Time: 20 minutes
Portion Size: 1 fillet of salmon with quinoa

Ingredients:
- 6 oz salmon fillet
- 1/2 cup quinoa, rinsed
- 1 cup of low-sodium chicken or vegetable broth
- 1 teaspoon dried dill
- 1 teaspoon lemon zest
- Lemon wedges for serving

Instructions:
1. Preheat oven to 375°F (190°C).
2. Season the salmon fillet with a pinch of salt and pepper.
3. Place salmon on a baking sheet lined with parchment paper and bake for about 12-15 minutes or until cooked through.
4. In a saucepan, combine quinoa, broth, dried dill, and lemon zest.

5. Bring to a boil, then reduce heat, cover, and simmer for 15-20 minutes or until quinoa is fluffy and liquid is absorbed.
6. Serve baked salmon on a bed of herbed quinoa with lemon wedges.

Nutritional Value (Approximate per serving):
Calories: 400
Total Fat: 18g
Saturated Fat: 3g
Cholesterol: 80mg
Sodium: 300mg
Total Carbohydrates: 30g
Dietary Fiber: 4g
Sugars: 2g
Protein: 30g

Lemon Herb Grilled Shrimp

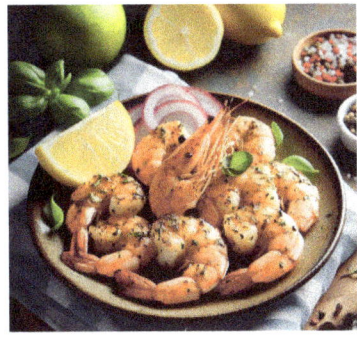

Preparation Time: 10 Minutes
Cooking Time: 5 minutes
Portion Size: 1 skewer of shrimp

Ingredients:
- 8 oz large shrimp, peeled and deveined
- Zest and juice of 1 lemon
- 1 tablespoon olive oil
- 1 clove garlic, minced
- 1 teaspoon dried herbs (thyme, rosemary, oregano)
- Salt and pepper to taste

Instructions:
1. In a bowl, whisk together lemon zest, lemon juice, olive oil, minced garlic, dried herbs, salt, and pepper.
2. Add shrimp to the marinade and let them sit for about 15-20 minutes.

3. The grill or grill pan is preheated over medium-high heat.
4. The shrimp is then grilled for 2-3 minutes per side or until they are opaque and cooked through.

Nutritional Value (Approximate per serving):
Calories: 150
Total Fat: 5g
Saturated Fat: 1g
Cholesterol: 150mg
Sodium: 250mg
Total Carbohydrates: 2g
Dietary Fiber: 0g
Sugars: 0g
Protein: 25g

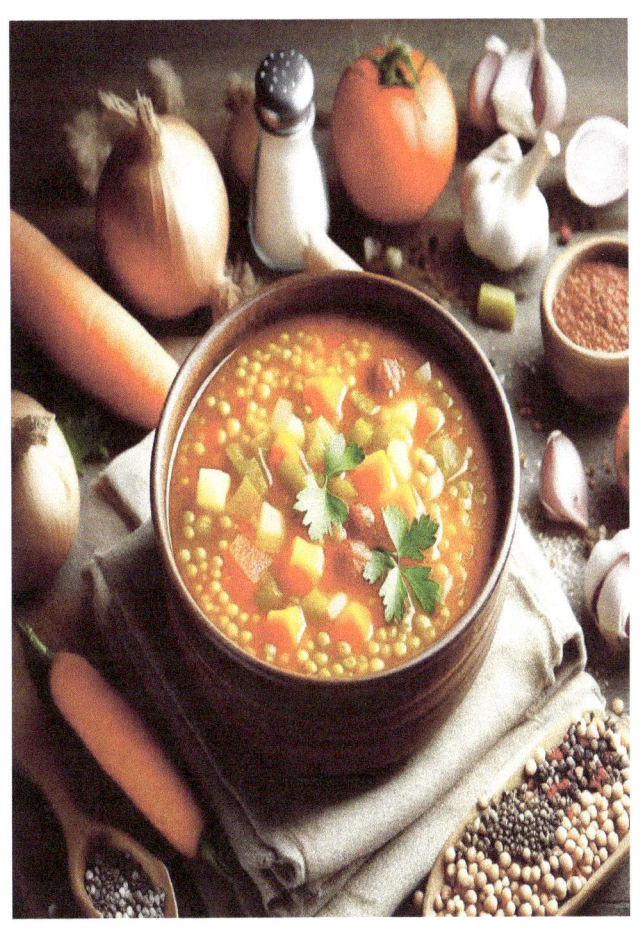

Chapter 4: Dinner Recipes

Creamy Broccoli Soup
Roasted Red Pepper Hummus
Herbed Baked Chicken
Teriyaki Salmon
Lemon Garlic Roasted Broccoli
Herb-Roasted Potatoes
Sweet Potato and Black Bean Hash
Lemon Herb Roasted Chicken Thighs
Roasted Vegetable Medley
Greek Chicken Souvlaki

Creamy Broccoli Soup

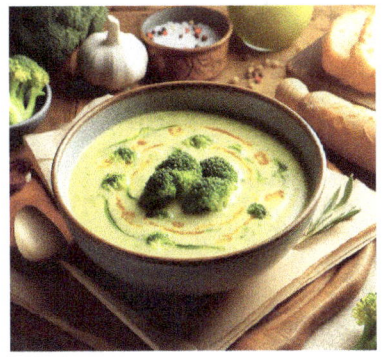

Preparation Time: 10 Minutes
Cooking Time: 20 minutes
Portion Size: 1 bowl

Ingredients:
- **2 cups broccoli florets**
- **1 small potato, peeled and diced**
- **1/2 onion, chopped**
- **2 cups low-sodium vegetable broth**
- **1/2 cup low-fat milk**
- **1/4 cup plain Greek yogurt**
- **Salt and pepper to taste**

Instructions:
1. In a pot, sauté chopped onion until translucent.
2. Add diced potato, broccoli florets, and vegetable broth.

3. Bring to a boil, then reduce heat and let it simmer until vegetables are tender.
4. Using an immersion blender, puree the soup until it is smooth.
5. Stir in low-fat milk and plain Greek yogurt. Season with salt and pepper.

Nutritional Value (Approximate per serving):
Calories: 150
Total Fat: 8g
Saturated Fat: 2g
Cholesterol: 10mg
Sodium: 400mg
Total Carbohydrates: 16g
Dietary Fiber: 4g
Sugars: 4g
Protein: 6g

Roasted Red Pepper Hummus

Preparation Time: 10 Minutes
Cooking Time: 20 minutes
Portion Size: 1/4 cup

Ingredients:
- 1 can (15 oz) low-sodium chickpeas, (they are to be rinsed and drained)
- 1/2 cup roasted red peppers, drained
- 2 tablespoons tahini
- 2 tablespoons lemon juice
- 1 clove garlic
- 1/4 teaspoon ground cumin
- Salt and pepper to taste

Instructions:
1. In a food processor, blend chickpeas, roasted red peppers, tahini, lemon juice, garlic, ground cumin, salt, and pepper until smooth.
2. A tablespoon of water can be added at a time until desired consistency is reached, if the hummus is too thick.
3. Serve the roasted red pepper hummus with sliced vegetables or whole wheat pita.

Nutritional Value (Approximate per serving):
Calories: 100
Total Fat: 7g
Saturated Fat: 1g
Cholesterol: 0mg
Sodium: 150mg
Total Carbohydrates: 8g
Dietary Fiber: 2g
Sugars: 2g
Protein: 2g

Herbed Baked Chicken

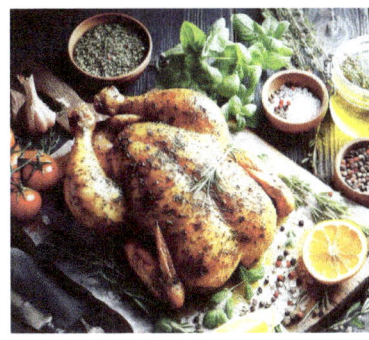

Preparation Time: 10 Minutes
Cooking Time: 30 minutes
Portion Size: 1 piece of chicken

Ingredients:
- 2 boneless, skinless chicken breasts
- 1 tablespoon olive oil
- 1 teaspoon of dried Italian herbs (any of oregano, basil or thyme will do)
- Salt and pepper to taste

Instructions:
1. Preheat the oven to 375°F (190°C).
2. Rub chicken breasts with olive oil, dried Italian herbs, salt, and pepper.
3. Place chicken on a baking sheet and bake for about 25-30 minutes or until cooked through.

Nutritional Value (Approximate per serving):
Calories: 250
Total Fat: 15g
Saturated Fat: 3g
Cholesterol: 80mg
Sodium: 350mg
Total Carbohydrates: 1g
Dietary Fiber: 0g
Sugars: 0g
Protein: 28g

Teriyaki Salmon

Preparation Time: 10 Minutes
Cooking Time: 15 minutes
Portion Size: 1 fillet of salmon

Ingredients:
- 2 salmon fillets
- 1/4 cup low-sodium teriyaki sauce
- 1 tablespoon honey
- 1 tablespoon rice vinegar
- 1 teaspoon grated ginger
- 1 clove garlic, minced
- 1/4 teaspoon sesame seeds

Instructions:
1. In a bowl, whisk together teriyaki sauce, honey, rice vinegar, grated ginger, and minced garlic.
2. Place salmon fillets in a shallow dish and pour the teriyaki marinade over them. Give them about 20-30 minutes to marinate.
3. The grill or grill pan is preheated over medium-high heat.
4. Grill salmon fillets for about 4-5 minutes per side or until they are cooked to your liking.

5. Sprinkle with sesame seeds before serving.

Nutritional Value (Approximate per serving):
Calories: 300
Total Fat: 12g
Saturated Fat: 2g
Cholesterol: 80mg
Sodium: 600mg
Total Carbohydrates: 18g
Dietary Fiber: 1g
Sugars: 15g
Protein: 28g

Lemon Garlic Roasted Broccoli

Preparation Time: 15 Minutes
Cooking Time: 15 minutes
Portion Size: 1 skewer

Ingredients:
- 2 cups broccoli florets
- Zest and juice of 1 lemon
- 2 tablespoons olive oil
- 2 cloves garlic, minced
- Salt and pepper to taste

Instructions:
1. Preheat the oven to 400°F (200°C).
2. In a bowl, toss broccoli florets with lemon zest, lemon juice, olive oil, minced garlic, salt, and pepper.
3. The broccoli is spread on a baking sheet in a single layer.
4. The broccoli is then roasted in the preheated oven for about 15-20 minutes or until it is tender and slightly crispy.

Nutritional Value (Approximate per serving):
Calories: 180
Total Fat: 5g
Saturated Fat: 1g
Cholesterol: 50mg
Sodium: 300mg
Total Carbohydrates: 12g
Dietary Fiber: 3g
Sugars: 6g
Protein: 20g

Herb-Roasted Potatoes

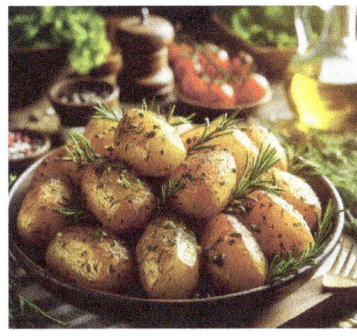

Preparation Time: 15 Minutes
Cooking Time: 30 minutes
Portion Size: 1/2 cup

Ingredients:
- 2 cups baby potatoes, halved
- 2 tablespoons olive oil
- 1 teaspoon of dried herbs (rosemary, thyme, oregano)
- Salt and pepper to taste

Instructions:
1. Preheat the oven to 400°F (200°C).
2. Toss halved baby potatoes with olive oil, dried herbs, salt, and pepper.
3. On a baking sheet, spread the potatoes in a single layer.

4. Roast in the preheated oven for about 20-25 minutes or until potatoes are golden and crispy.

Nutritional Value (Approximate per serving):
Calories: 150
Total Fat: 5g
Saturated Fat: 1g
Cholesterol: 0mg
Sodium: 250mg
Total Carbohydrates: 25g
Dietary Fiber: 3g
Sugars: 2g
Protein: 2g

Sweet Potato and Black Bean Hash

Preparation Time: 15 Minutes
Cooking Time: 20 minutes
Portion Size: 1 serving

Ingredients:

- 1 medium-sized sweet potato (peeled and diced)
- 1/2 cup canned low-sodium black beans, (they are to be rinsed and drained)
- 1/2 red bell pepper, diced
- 1/4 red onion, diced
- 1/2 teaspoon ground cumin
- 1/4 teaspoon smoked paprika
- Salt and pepper to taste
- 2 eggs (optional)

Instructions:

1. In a skillet, sauté sweet potato, black beans, red bell pepper, and red onion until sweet potato is cooked and slightly crispy.
2. Add ground cumin, smoked paprika, salt, and pepper, and stir to combine.

3. If desired, create two wells in the hash and crack eggs into them. Cover the skillet, cooking until the eggs are cooked to your preference.

Nutritional Value (Approximate per serving):
Calories: 300
Total Fat: 8g
Saturated Fat: 1g
Cholesterol: 0mg
Sodium: 400mg
Total Carbohydrates: 50g
Dietary Fiber: 12g
Sugars: 8g
Protein: 10g

Lemon Herb Roasted Chicken Thighs

Preparation Time: 10 Minutes
Cooking Time: 35 minutes
Portion Size: 1 chicken thigh

Ingredients:
- 4 bone-in, skin-on chicken thighs
- Zest and juice of 1 lemon
- 2 tablespoons olive oil
- 1 teaspoon dried herbs (thyme, rosemary, oregano)
- 2 cloves garlic, minced
- Salt and pepper to taste

Instructions:
1. Preheat the oven to 375°F (190°C).
2. In a bowl, whisk together lemon zest, lemon juice, olive oil, dried herbs, minced garlic, salt, and pepper.
3. The chicken thighs are placed on a baking sheet lined with parchment paper.
4. Brush the lemon herb mixture over the chicken thighs.

5. Bake for about 30-35 minutes or until chicken is cooked through and skin is crispy.

Nutritional Value (Approximate per serving):
Calories: 250
Total Fat: 15g
Saturated Fat: 4g
Cholesterol: 130mg
Sodium: 350mg
Total Carbohydrates: 1g
Dietary Fiber: 0g
Sugars: 0g
Protein: 25g

Roasted Vegetable Medley

Preparation Time: 10 Minutes
Cooking Time: 20 minutes
Portion Size: 1 cup

Ingredients:
- 2 cups mixed vegetables (zucchini, bell peppers, carrots, eggplant), chopped
- 1 tablespoon olive oil
- 1 teaspoon dried herbs (thyme, rosemary, oregano)
- Salt and pepper to taste

Instructions:
1. Preheat the oven to 400°F (200°C).
2. Toss chopped vegetables with olive oil, dried herbs, salt, and pepper.
3. The vegetables are spread in a single layer on a baking sheet.
4. Roast in the preheated oven for 20-25 minutes or until vegetables are tender and slightly caramelized.

Nutritional Value (Approximate per serving):
Calories: 100
Total Fat: 5g
Saturated Fat: 1g
Cholesterol: 0mg
Sodium: 200mg
Total Carbohydrates: 15g
Dietary Fiber: 4g
Sugars:6g
Protein: 2g

Greek Chicken Souvlaki

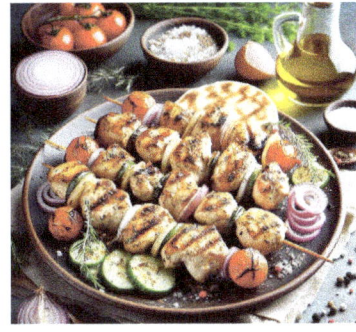

Preparation Time: 15 Minutes
Cooking Time: 15 minutes
Portion Size: 1 skewer of chicken

Ingredients:
- 8 oz boneless, skinless chicken breast (cut it into cubes)
- 1/4 cup plain Greek yogurt
- Juice of 1 lemon
- 1 teaspoon dried oregano
- 2 cloves garlic, minced
- Salt and pepper to taste

Instructions:
1. In a bowl, mix plain Greek yogurt, lemon juice, dried oregano, minced garlic, salt, and pepper.
2. Add chicken cubes to the marinade and let them marinate for about 20-30 minutes.

3. The grill or grill pan is preheated over medium-high heat.
4. Thread marinated chicken cubes onto skewers and grill for about 8-10 minutes, turning occasionally, until chicken is cooked through.

Nutritional Value (Approximate per serving):
Calories: 250
Total Fat: 10g
Saturated Fat: 2g
Cholesterol: 85mg
Sodium: 400mg
Total Carbohydrates: 8g
Dietary Fiber: 2g
Sugars: 4g
Protein: 30g

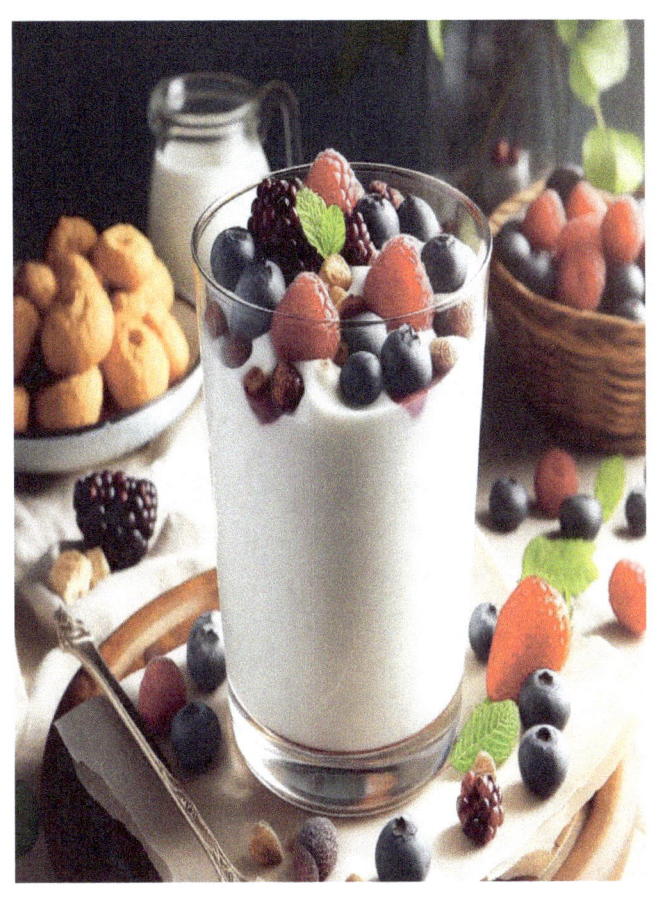

Chapter 5: Desserts

Mixed Berry Chia Pudding
Baked Apple with Cinnamon
Vanilla Banana "Ice Cream"
Chia Seed Pudding with Mango
Poached Pears with Cinnamon
Coconut Rice Pudding
Mango Sorbet
Banana Oat Cookies
Rice Pudding with Cinnamon and Raisins
Watermelon Sorbet

Mixed Berry Chia Pudding

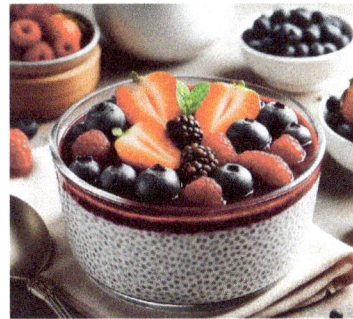

Preparation Time: 10 Minutes
Cooking Time: 0 minutes (refrigeration required)
Portion Size: 1 serving

Ingredients:
- 2 tbsp chia seeds
- 1 cup of almond milk (other non-dairy milk alternatives are great too)
- 1/2 cup of mixed berries, including blueberries, strawberries, and raspberries)

Instructions:
1. Mix chia seeds and almond milk in a bowl, stirring the mixture well and refrigerating it for at least 2 hours or overnight.
2. Before serving, give the chia pudding a good stir to ensure the seeds are evenly distributed and have absorbed the liquid.

3. Top with mixed berries and enjoy.

Nutritional Value (Approximate per serving):
Calories: 200
Total Fat: 8g
Saturated Fat: 2g
Cholesterol: 0mg
Sodium: 50mg
Total Carbohydrates: 25g
Dietary Fiber: 8g
Sugars: 12g
Protein: 6g

Baked Apple with Cinnamon

Preparation Time: 10 Minutes
Cooking Time: 25 minutes
Portion Size: 1 baked apple

Ingredients:
- 1 medium apple
- 1 tsp cinnamon
- 1 tsp honey (optional)

Instructions:
1. Preheat the oven to 350°F (175°C).
2. Core the apple and place it in a baking dish.
3. Sprinkle cinnamon over the apple and drizzle with honey if desired.
4. Bake for 25 minutes or until the apple is tender.
5. Serve warm.

Nutritional Value (Approximate per serving):
Calories: 150
Total Fat: 1g
Saturated Fat: 0g
Cholesterol: 0mg

Sodium: 0mg
Total Carbohydrates: 40g
Dietary Fiber: 6g
Sugars: 29g
Protein: 1g

Vanilla Banana "Ice Cream"

Preparation Time: 5 Minutes
Cooking Time: 0 minutes (freezing required)
Portion Size: 1 serving

Ingredients:
- 1 ripe banana, frozen
- 1/2 tsp vanilla extract

Instructions:
1. Peel and slice the frozen banana.
2. Place the banana slices in a food processor or blender.
3. Add vanilla extract.
4. Blend until smooth and creamy, resembling the texture of ice cream.
5. Serve immediately as soft-serve or freeze for an additional hour for a firmer texture.

Nutritional Value (Approximate per serving):
Calories: 100
Total Fat: 0g
Saturated Fat: 0g
Cholesterol: 0mg

Sodium: 0mg
Total Carbohydrates: 25g
Dietary Fiber: 3g
Sugars: 14g
Protein: 1g

Chia Seed Pudding with Mango

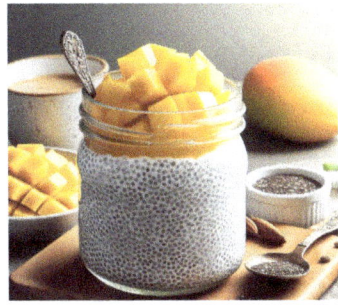

Preparation Time: 10 Minutes

Cooking Time: 0 minutes (refrigeration required)

Portion Size: 1 serving

Ingredients:
- 2 tbsp chia seeds
- 1/2 cup unsweetened almond milk (other non-dairy alternatives can also be used)
- 1/2 cup diced mango

Instructions:
1. Combine chia seeds and almond milk, in a bowl, stirring the mixture well and refrigerating it for at least 2 hours or overnight.
2. Before serving, give the chia pudding a good stir to ensure the seeds are evenly distributed and have absorbed the liquid.
3. Top with diced mango and enjoy.

Nutritional Value (Approximate per serving):
Calories: 150
Total Fat: 5g
Saturated Fat: 0.5g
Cholesterol: 0mg
Sodium: 0mg
Total Carbohydrates: 25g
Dietary Fiber: 10g
Sugars: 15g
Protein: 3g

Poached Pears with Cinnamon

Preparation Time: 10 Minutes
Cooking Time: 20 minutes
Portion Size: 1 poached pear

Ingredients:
- 1 pear, peeled and cored
- 1 cinnamon stick
- 1 cup water
- 1 tsp honey (optional)

Instructions:
1. In a saucepan, combine water and cinnamon stick. Bring to a simmer.
2. Add the peeled and cored pear to the simmering water. Cover and poach for about 15-20 minutes or until the pear is tender.
3. Remove the pear from the liquid and let it cool slightly.
4. Drizzle with honey if desired and serve warm.

Nutritional Value (Approximate per serving):
Calories: 120
Total Fat: 0g
Saturated Fat: 0g
Cholesterol: 0mg
Sodium: 5mg
Total Carbohydrates: 32g
Dietary Fiber: 5g
Sugars: 21g
Protein: 1g

Coconut Rice Pudding

Preparation Time: 5 Minutes
Cooking Time: 25 minutes
Portion Size: 1 serving

Ingredients:
- **1/4 cup Arborio rice**
- **1 cup unsweetened coconut milk**
- **1/4 cup sugar**
- **1/2 tsp vanilla extract**
- **Pinch of salt**
- **Ground cinnamon for garnish**

Instructions:
1. Rinse the Arborio rice under cold water and drain.
2. In a saucepan, combine the rice, coconut milk, sugar, vanilla extract, and salt. Let it simmer over medium heat.
3. Reduce the heat to low and let the mixture cook, stirring occasionally, for about 20-25 minutes or until the rice is tender and the mixture has thickened.
4. The mixture is removed from heat and allowed to cool slightly.

5. Serve warm or chilled, garnished with a sprinkle of ground cinnamon.

Nutritional Value (Approximate per serving):
Calories: 180
Total Fat: 5g
Saturated Fat: 4g
Cholesterol: 0mg
Sodium: 10mg
Total Carbohydrates: 30g
Dietary Fiber: 1g
Sugars: 15g
Protein: 3g

Mango Sorbet

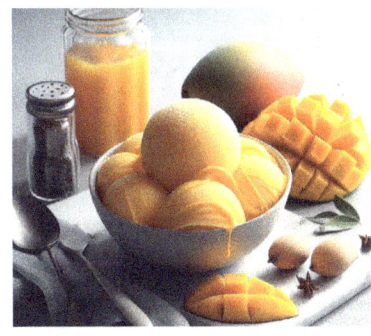

Preparation Time: 10 Minutes
Cooking Time: 0 minutes (freezing required)
Portion Size: 1 serving

Ingredients:
- 1 cup diced mango (fresh or frozen)
- 1 tsp lime juice
- 1 tsp honey (optional)

Instructions:
1. If using fresh mango, dice it and freeze for at least 1 hour. If using frozen mango, thaw slightly.
2. Place the diced mango, lime juice, and honey (if using) in a blender or food processor.
3. Blend until smooth and creamy.
4. Serve immediately as soft sorbet or freeze for an additional hour for a firmer texture.

Nutritional Value (Approximate per serving):
Calories: 80
Total Fat: 0g
Saturated Fat: 0g
Cholesterol: 0mg
Sodium: 0mg
Total Carbohydrates: 20g
Dietary Fiber: 2g
Sugars: 18g
Protein: 1g

Banana Oat Cookies

Preparation Time: 10 Minutes
Cooking Time: 0 minutes (freezing required)
Portion Size: 1 serving

Ingredients:
- 1 ripe banana, mashed
- 1 cup rolled oats
- 1/4 cup unsweetened applesauce
- 1/4 cup chopped walnuts
- 1/2 tsp vanilla extract
- 1/2 tsp ground cinnamon
- Pinch of salt

Instructions:
1. The oven is preheated to 350°F (175°C) and a baking sheet is lined with parchment paper.
2. In a bowl, combine mashed banana, rolled oats, applesauce, chopped walnuts, vanilla extract, ground cinnamon, and a pinch of salt. Mix well.
3. Drop spoonfuls of the mixture onto the prepared baking sheet to form cookies.

4. Bake for 15-18 minutes or until the cookies are golden and firm.
5. Allow the cookies to cool before enjoying.

Nutritional Value (Approximate per serving):
Calories: 120
Total Fat: 3g
Saturated Fat: 0.5g
Cholesterol: 0mg
Sodium: 5mg
Total Carbohydrates: 22g
Dietary Fiber: 2g
Sugars: 7g
Protein: 3g

Rice Pudding with Cinnamon and Raisins

Preparation Time: 10 Minutes
Cooking Time: 30 minutes
Portion Size: 1 serving

Ingredients:
- 1/4 cup Arborio rice
- 1 cup low-fat milk
- 1 tbsp sugar
- 1/2 tsp vanilla extract
- 1/2 tsp ground cinnamon
- 1 tbsp raisins

Instructions:
1. Rinse the Arborio rice under cold water and drain.
2. In a saucepan, combine the rice and milk. The mixture is brought to a simmer over medium heat.
3. Reduce the heat to low and let the mixture cook, stirring occasionally, for about 20-25 minutes or until the rice is tender and the mixture has thickened.

4. Stir in sugar, vanilla extract, ground cinnamon, and raisins. Cook for an additional 5 minutes.
5. Remove from heat, allowing it to cool slightly before serving.

Nutritional Value (Approximate per serving):
Calories: 180
Total Fat: 3g
Saturated Fat: 1.5g
Cholesterol: 5mg
Sodium: 25mg
Total Carbohydrates: 34g
Dietary Fiber: 0g
Sugars: 18g
Protein: 3g

Watermelon Sorbet

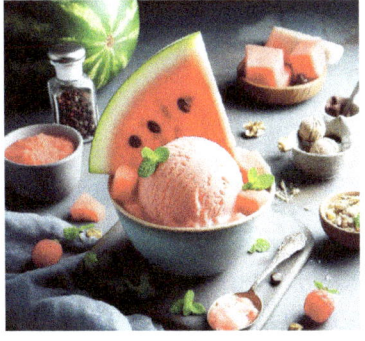

Preparation Time:
10 Minutes
Cooking Time: 0
minutes (freezing
required)
Portion Size: 1
serving

Ingredients:
- **1 cup diced watermelon**
- **1 tsp lime juice**
- **1 tsp honey (optional)**

Instructions:
1. Place the diced watermelon, lime juice, and honey (if using) in a blender or food processor.
2. Blend until smooth and creamy.
3. Serve immediately as soft sorbet or freeze for an additional hour for a firmer texture.

Nutritional Value (Approximate per serving):
Calories: 70
Total Fat: 0g
Saturated Fat: 0g
Cholesterol: 0mg
Sodium: 0mg
Total Carbohydrates: 18g
Dietary Fiber: 1g
Sugars: 14g
Protein: 1g

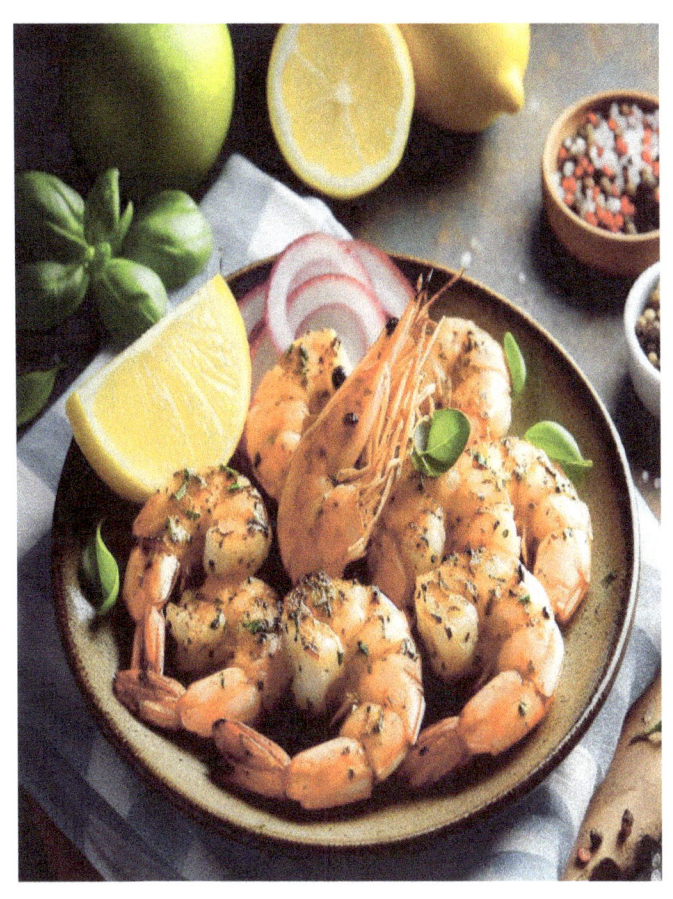

14-Day Kidney-Friendly Meal Plan

Day 1:
Breakfast: Creamy Oatmeal with Fresh Berries
Lunch: Greek Chicken Souvlaki with Mixed Green Salad
Dinner: Lemon Herb Grilled Shrimp with Roasted Vegetable Medley
Dessert: Mixed Berry Chia Pudding

Day 2:
Breakfast: Spinach and Mushroom Frittata
Lunch: Quinoa Stuffed Bell Peppers
Dinner: Teriyaki Salmon with Steamed Broccoli
Dessert: Baked Apple with Cinnamon

Day 3:
Breakfast: Greek Yogurt Parfait with Mixed Berries
Lunch: Italian Bean Salad with Grilled Chicken
Dinner: Mushroom and Spinach Stuffed Chicken Breast with Herb-Roasted Potatoes
Dessert: Vanilla Banana "Ice Cream"

Day 4:
Breakfast: Veggie and Brown Rice Stir-Fry
Lunch: Caprese Salad with Whole Wheat Roll

Dinner: Roasted Beet and Goat Cheese Salad with Lemon Garlic Roasted Broccoli
Dessert: Mango Sorbet

Day 5:
Breakfast: Mixed Berry Smoothie Bowl
Lunch: Turkey and Vegetable Stir-Fry with Brown Rice
Dinner: Zucchini Noodles with Pesto and Grilled Shrimp
Dessert: Chia Seed Pudding with Mango

Day 6:
Breakfast: Sweet Potato and Black Bean Hash
Lunch: Greek Chickpea Salad with Tuna
Dinner: Honey Mustard Glazed Salmon with Asparagus
Dessert: Poached Pears with Cinnamon

Day 7:
Breakfast: Scrambled Eggs with Sautéed Spinach and Tomatoes
Lunch: Lentil and Vegetable Soup with Whole Grain Bread
Dinner: Herb-Roasted Potatoes with Lemon Herb Roasted Chicken Thighs
Dessert: Coconut Rice Pudding

Day 8:

Breakfast: Greek Yogurt Parfait with Mixed Berries

Lunch: Turkey Meatballs with Marinara Sauce and Roasted Vegetable Medley

Dinner: Lemon Garlic Roasted Chicken Thighs with Quinoa and Vegetable Stuffed Bell Peppers

Dessert: Mango Sorbet

Day 9:

Breakfast: Mixed Berry Smoothie Bowl

Lunch: Greek Chickpea Salad with Grilled Chicken

Dinner: Herbed Baked Chicken with Lemon Herb Grilled Shrimp

Dessert: Banana Oat Cookies

Day 10:

Breakfast: Spinach and Mushroom Frittata

Lunch: Caprese Salad with Whole Wheat Roll

Dinner: Roasted Beet and Goat Cheese Salad with Lemon Garlic Roasted Broccoli

Dessert: Rice Pudding with Cinnamon and Raisins

Day 11:

Breakfast: Veggie and Brown Rice Stir-Fry

Lunch: Italian Bean Salad with Grilled Turkey Breast

Dinner: Mushroom and Spinach Stuffed Chicken Breast with Herb-Roasted Potatoes

Dessert: Watermelon Sorbet

Day 12:
Breakfast: Sweet Potato and Black Bean Hash
Lunch: Mediterranean Chickpea Salad with Tuna
Dinner: Honey Mustard Glazed Salmon with Asparagus
Dessert: Vanilla Banana "Ice Cream"

Day 13:
Breakfast: Scrambled Eggs with Sautéed Spinach and Tomatoes
Lunch: Lentil and Vegetable Soup with Whole Grain Bread
Dinner: Teriyaki Salmon with Steamed Broccoli
Dessert: Mixed Berry Chia Pudding

Day 14
Breakfast: Creamy Oatmeal with Fresh Berries
Lunch: Greek Chicken Souvlaki with Mixed Green Salad
Dinner: Zucchini Noodles with Pesto and Grilled Shrimp
Dessert: Coconut Rice Pudding

Conclusion

As we come to the end of this book, I want to take a moment to say a heartfelt thank you for joining me on this journey. Navigating Stage 3 kidney disease isn't easy, and your commitment to learning about kidney-friendly diets is truly admirable.

From the delicious recipes to the thoughtfully crafted meal plans, I hope you've found inspiration and practical tips to make your culinary experiences both enjoyable and health-conscious. Remember, you're not alone in this – every meal you prepare is a step towards nurturing your well-being.

As you close the chapters of this book, I encourage you to carry forward the knowledge and recipes with you. May they serve as your companions in the kitchen, reminding you that mindful eating is a powerful tool in managing your health.

Here's to your journey of flavors, well-being, and savoring every bite. Keep exploring, keep experimenting, and most importantly, keep taking care of yourself. Thank you for being a part of this, and may your path ahead be filled with nourishment and joy.

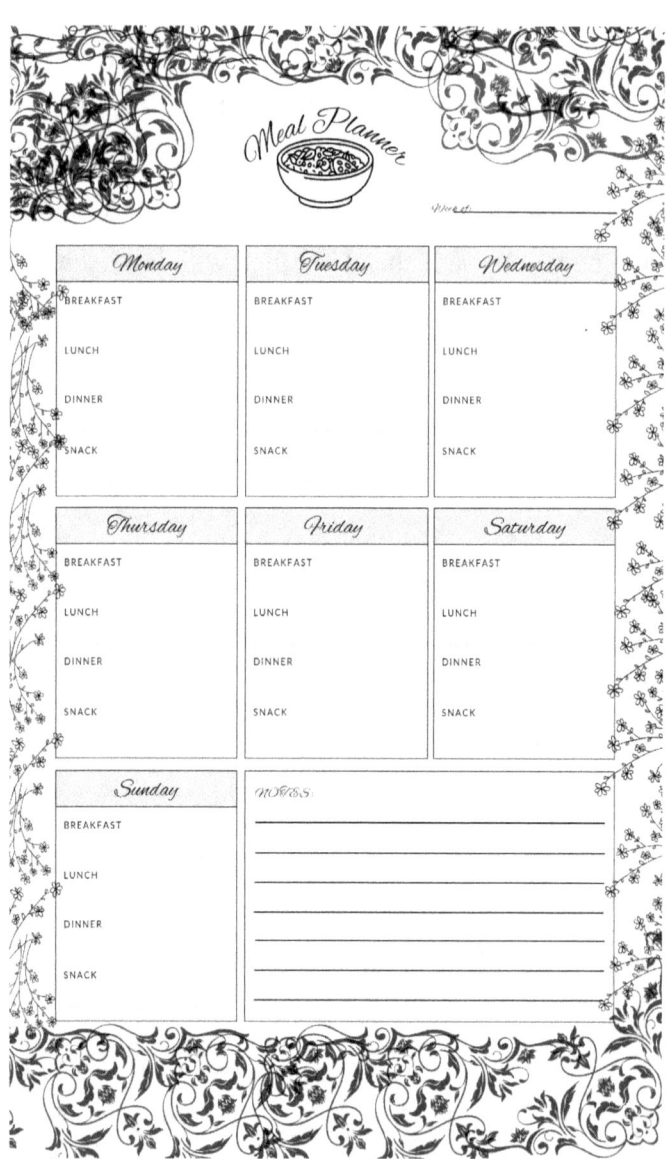

Meal Planner

Week: _____

Monday
BREAKFAST

LUNCH

DINNER

SNACK

Tuesday
BREAKFAST

LUNCH

DINNER

SNACK

Wednesday
BREAKFAST

LUNCH

DINNER

SNACK

Thursday
BREAKFAST

LUNCH

DINNER

SNACK

Friday
BREAKFAST

LUNCH

DINNER

SNACK

Saturday
BREAKFAST

LUNCH

DINNER

SNACK

Sunday
BREAKFAST

LUNCH

DINNER

SNACK

NOTES:
_____
_____
_____
_____
_____
_____

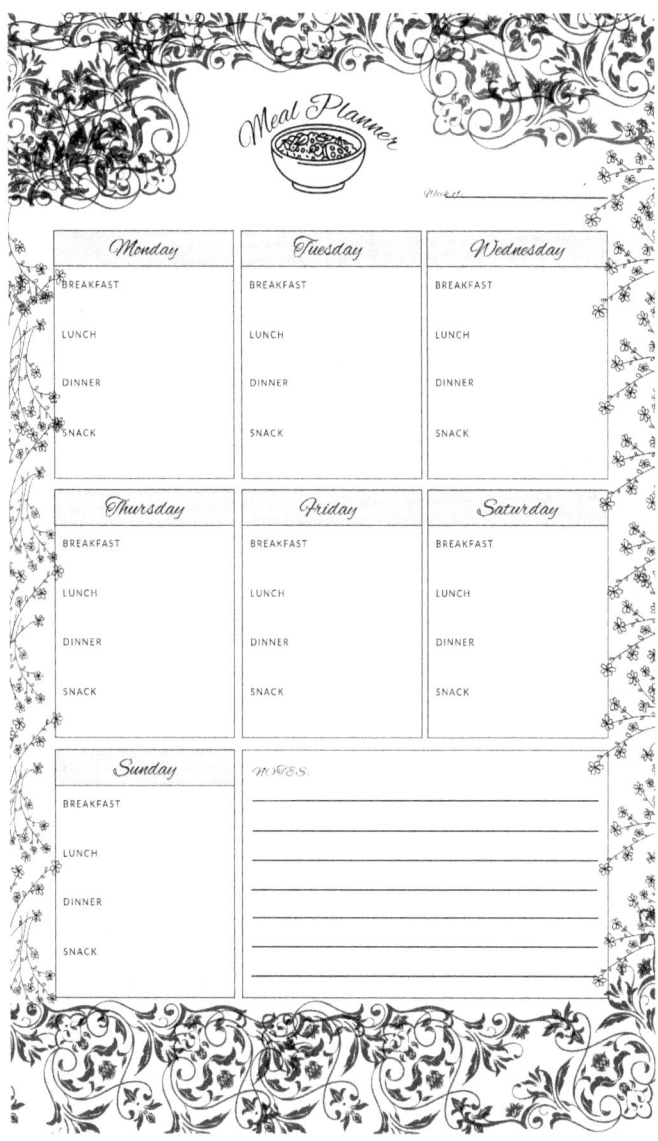

Meal Planner

Week: _____

Monday
BREAKFAST

LUNCH

DINNER

SNACK

Tuesday
BREAKFAST

LUNCH

DINNER

SNACK

Wednesday
BREAKFAST

LUNCH

DINNER

SNACK

Thursday
BREAKFAST

LUNCH

DINNER

SNACK

Friday
BREAKFAST

LUNCH

DINNER

SNACK

Saturday
BREAKFAST

LUNCH

DINNER

SNACK

Sunday
BREAKFAST

LUNCH

DINNER

SNACK

NOTES:
_____
_____
_____
_____
_____
_____

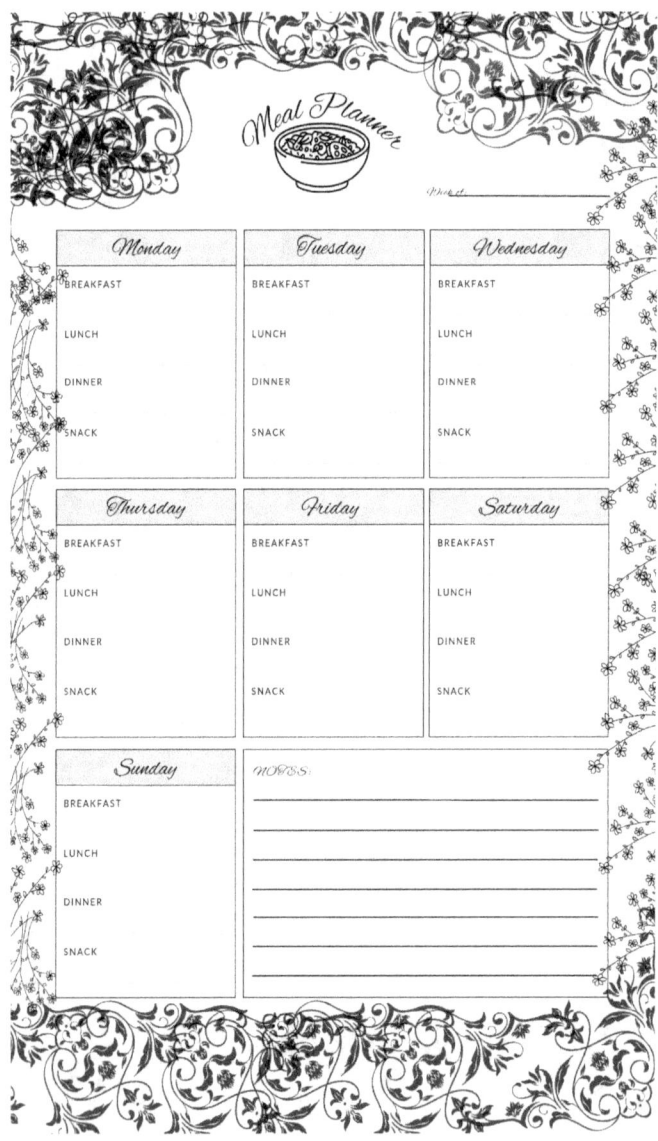

Meal Planner

Week: _____

Monday
BREAKFAST

LUNCH

DINNER

SNACK

Tuesday
BREAKFAST

LUNCH

DINNER

SNACK

Wednesday
BREAKFAST

LUNCH

DINNER

SNACK

Thursday
BREAKFAST

LUNCH

DINNER

SNACK

Friday
BREAKFAST

LUNCH

DINNER

SNACK

Saturday
BREAKFAST

LUNCH

DINNER

SNACK

Sunday
BREAKFAST

LUNCH

DINNER

SNACK

NOTES:
_____
_____
_____
_____
_____
_____
_____

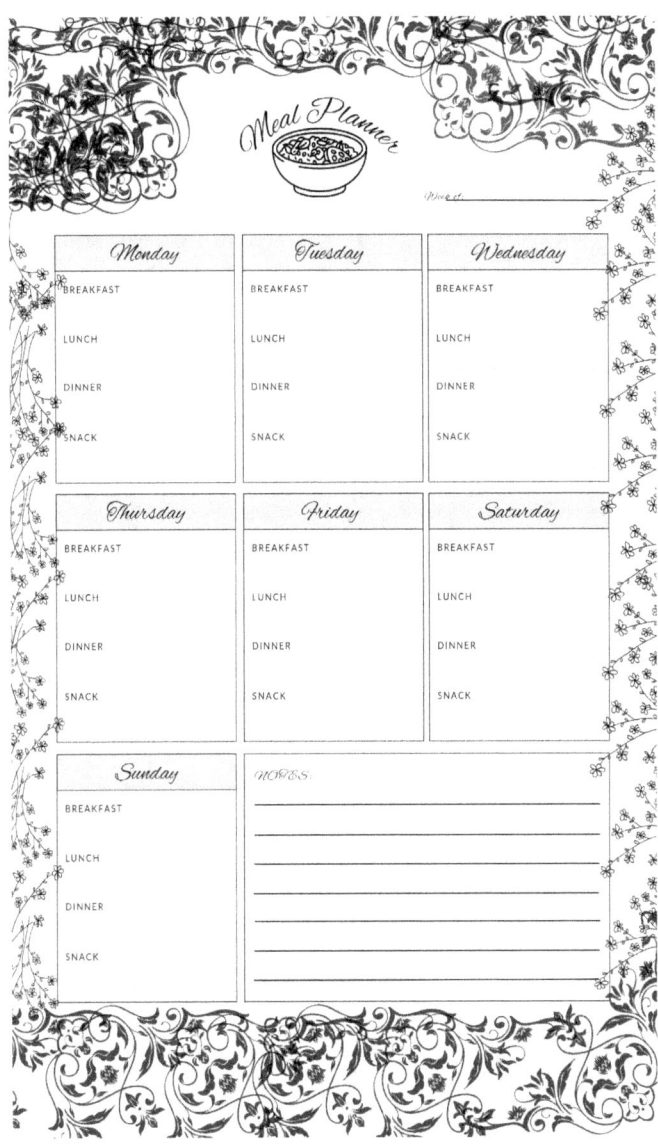

Meal Planner

Week:

Monday
BREAKFAST

LUNCH

DINNER

SNACK

Tuesday
BREAKFAST

LUNCH

DINNER

SNACK

Wednesday
BREAKFAST

LUNCH

DINNER

SNACK

Thursday
BREAKFAST

LUNCH

DINNER

SNACK

Friday
BREAKFAST

LUNCH

DINNER

SNACK

Saturday
BREAKFAST

LUNCH

DINNER

SNACK

Sunday
BREAKFAST

LUNCH

DINNER

SNACK

NOTES:

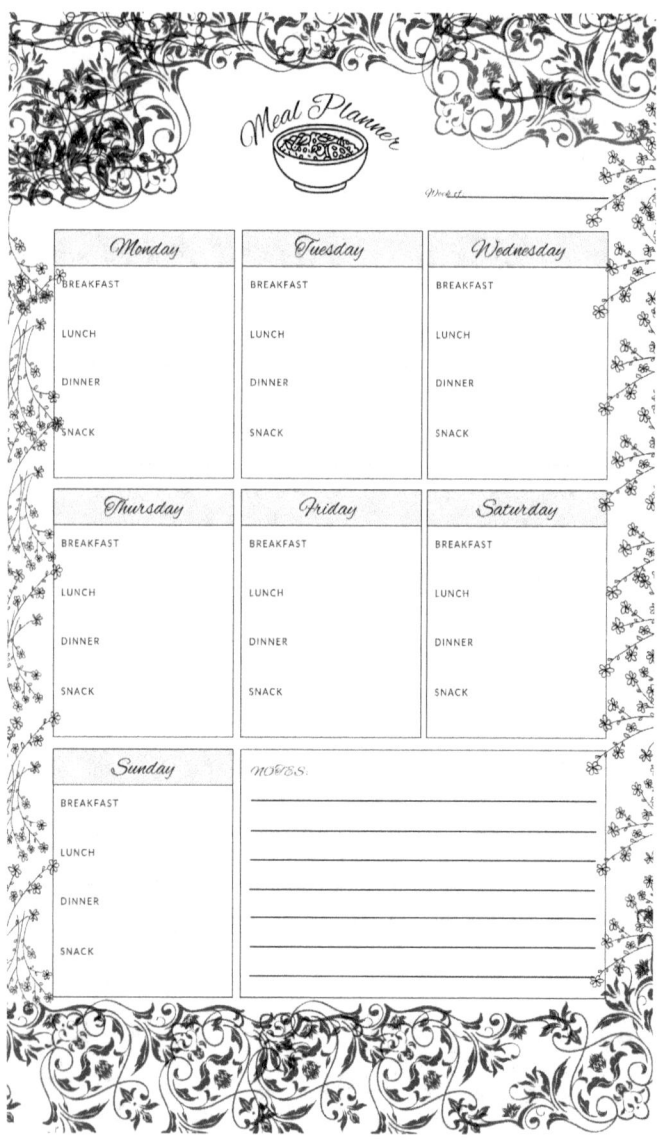

Meal Planner

Market _____

Monday
BREAKFAST

LUNCH

DINNER

SNACK

Tuesday
BREAKFAST

LUNCH

DINNER

SNACK

Wednesday
BREAKFAST

LUNCH

DINNER

SNACK

Thursday
BREAKFAST

LUNCH

DINNER

SNACK

Friday
BREAKFAST

LUNCH

DINNER

SNACK

Saturday
BREAKFAST

LUNCH

DINNER

SNACK

Sunday
BREAKFAST

LUNCH

DINNER

SNACK

NOTES
_____
_____
_____
_____
_____
_____

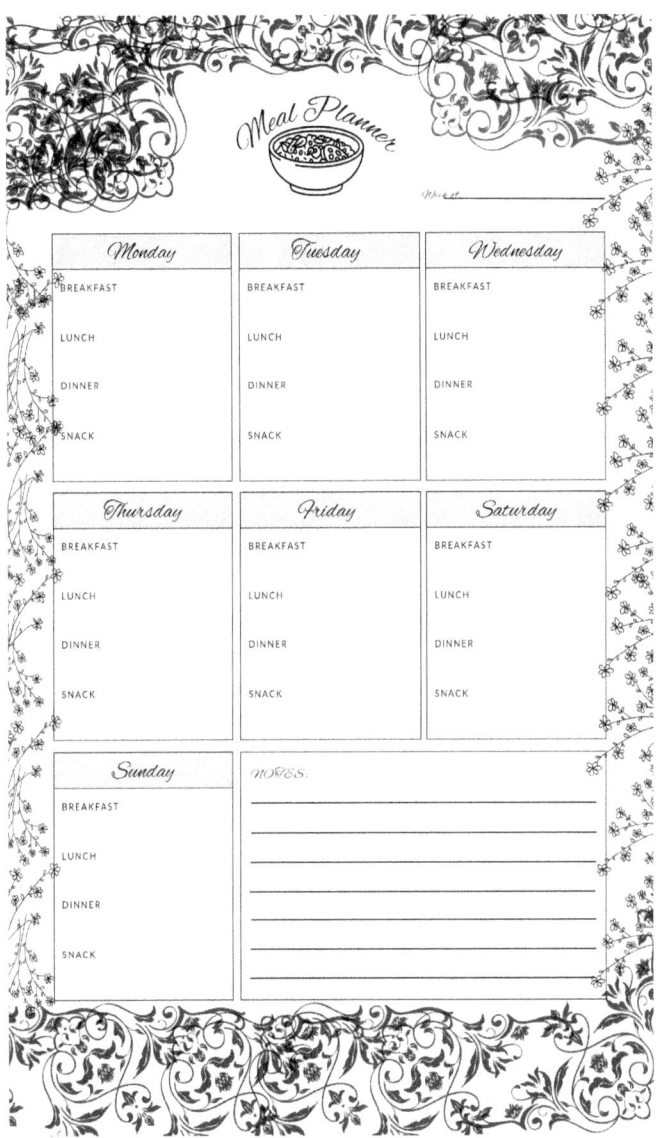

Meal Planner

Week:

Monday
BREAKFAST

LUNCH

DINNER

SNACK

Tuesday
BREAKFAST

LUNCH

DINNER

SNACK

Wednesday
BREAKFAST

LUNCH

DINNER

SNACK

Thursday
BREAKFAST

LUNCH

DINNER

SNACK

Friday
BREAKFAST

LUNCH

DINNER

SNACK

Saturday
BREAKFAST

LUNCH

DINNER

SNACK

Sunday
BREAKFAST

LUNCH

DINNER

SNACK

NOTES:

_____

_____

_____

_____

_____

116

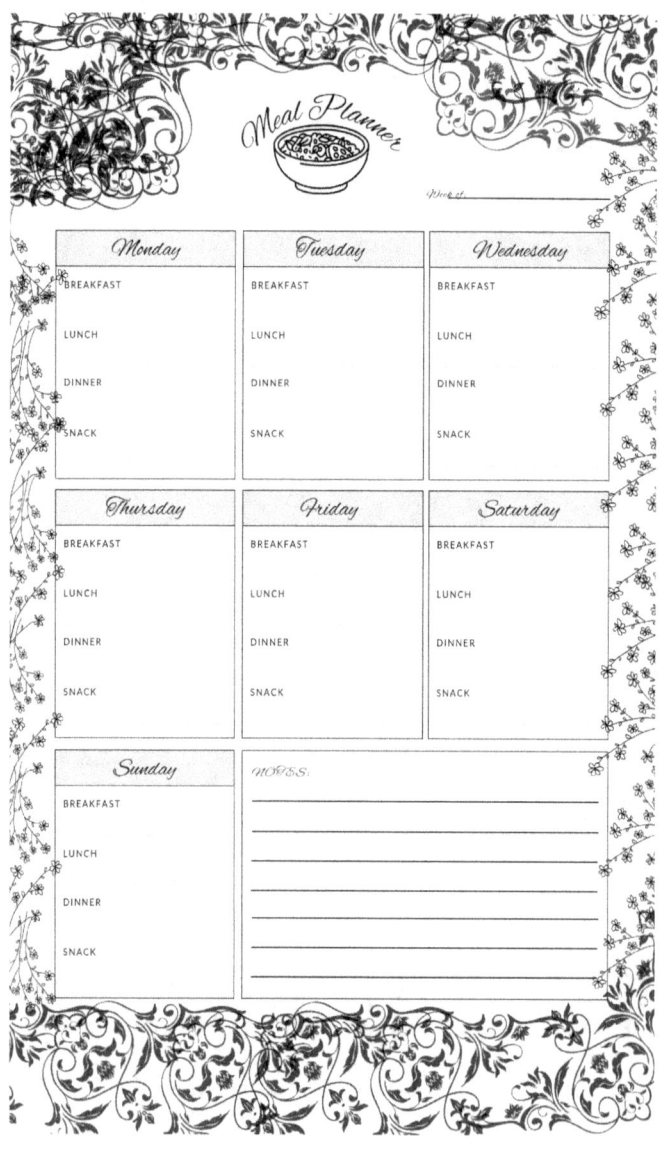

Meal Planner

Week of _____

Monday
BREAKFAST

LUNCH

DINNER

SNACK

Tuesday
BREAKFAST

LUNCH

DINNER

SNACK

Wednesday
BREAKFAST

LUNCH

DINNER

SNACK

Thursday
BREAKFAST

LUNCH

DINNER

SNACK

Friday
BREAKFAST

LUNCH

DINNER

SNACK

Saturday
BREAKFAST

LUNCH

DINNER

SNACK

Sunday
BREAKFAST

LUNCH

DINNER

SNACK

Notes
_____
_____
_____
_____
_____
_____

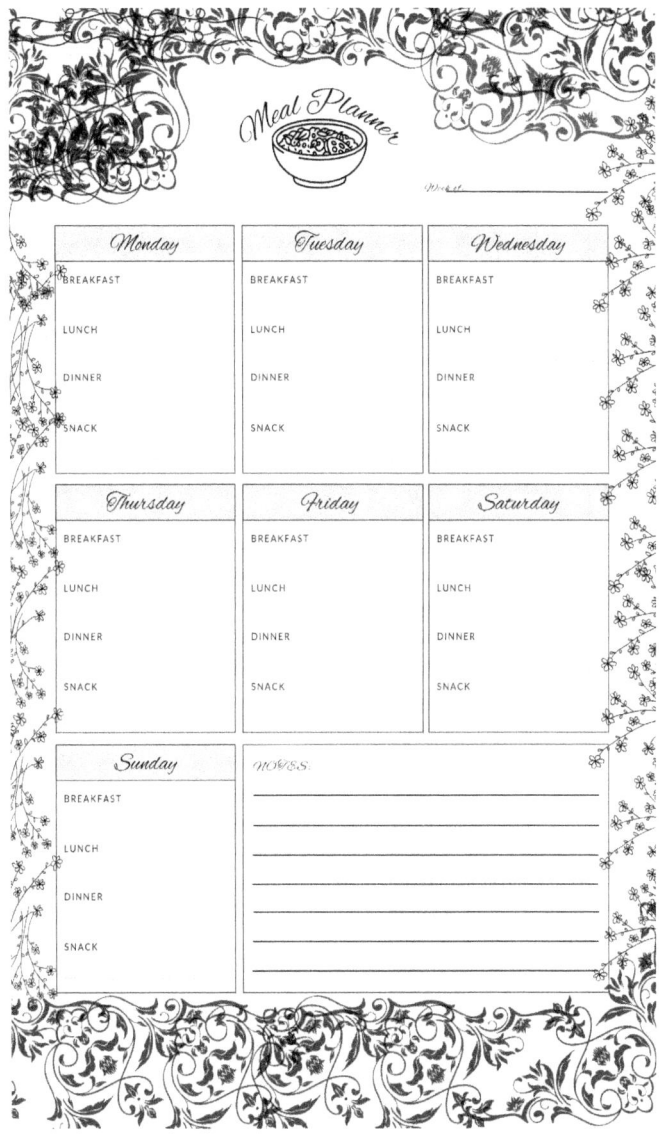

Meal Planner

Week: _____

Monday
BREAKFAST

LUNCH

DINNER

SNACK

Tuesday
BREAKFAST

LUNCH

DINNER

SNACK

Wednesday
BREAKFAST

LUNCH

DINNER

SNACK

Thursday
BREAKFAST

LUNCH

DINNER

SNACK

Friday
BREAKFAST

LUNCH

DINNER

SNACK

Saturday
BREAKFAST

LUNCH

DINNER

SNACK

Sunday
BREAKFAST

LUNCH

DINNER

SNACK

NOTES:
_____
_____
_____
_____
_____
_____
_____

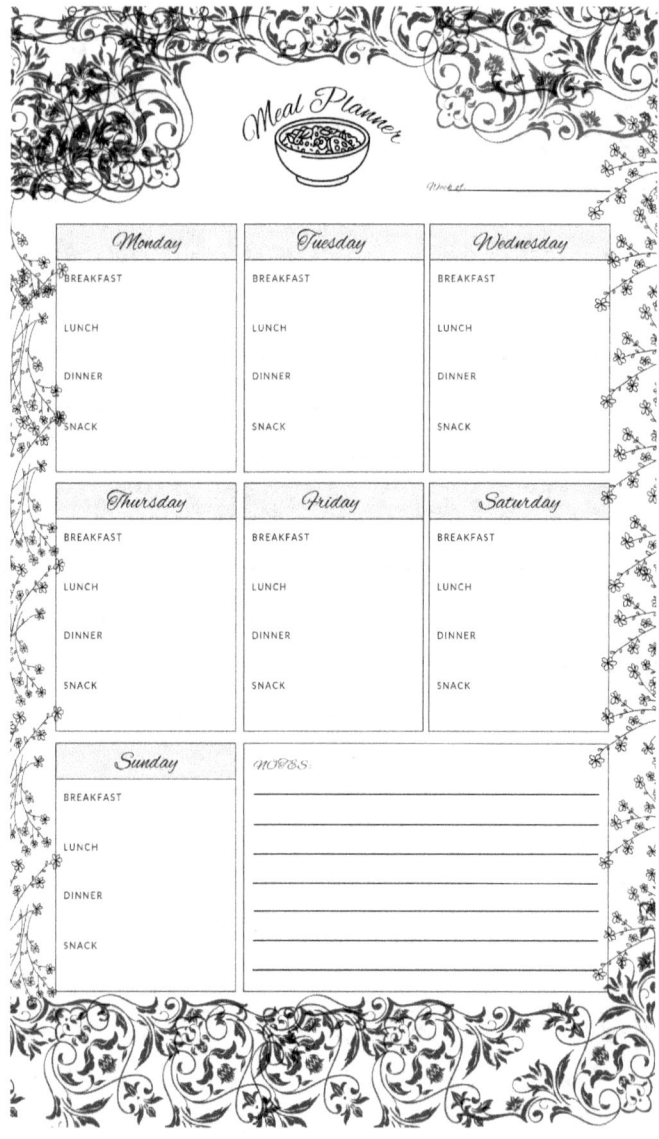

Meal Planner

Week of: _____

Monday
BREAKFAST

LUNCH

DINNER

SNACK

Tuesday
BREAKFAST

LUNCH

DINNER

SNACK

Wednesday
BREAKFAST

LUNCH

DINNER

SNACK

Thursday
BREAKFAST

LUNCH

DINNER

SNACK

Friday
BREAKFAST

LUNCH

DINNER

SNACK

Saturday
BREAKFAST

LUNCH

DINNER

SNACK

Sunday
BREAKFAST

LUNCH

DINNER

SNACK

Notes:
_____
_____
_____
_____
_____
_____

119

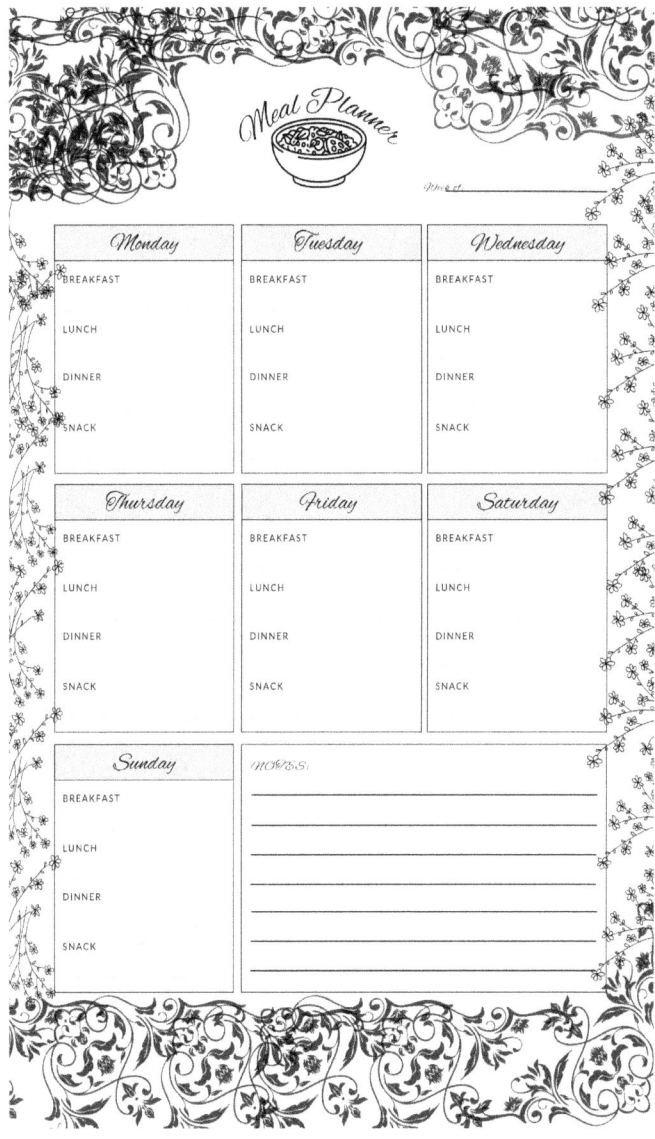

Meal Planner

Week of: _____

Monday
BREAKFAST

LUNCH

DINNER

SNACK

Tuesday
BREAKFAST

LUNCH

DINNER

SNACK

Wednesday
BREAKFAST

LUNCH

DINNER

SNACK

Thursday
BREAKFAST

LUNCH

DINNER

SNACK

Friday
BREAKFAST

LUNCH

DINNER

SNACK

Saturday
BREAKFAST

LUNCH

DINNER

SNACK

Sunday
BREAKFAST

LUNCH

DINNER

SNACK

NOTES:
_____
_____
_____
_____
_____
_____
_____

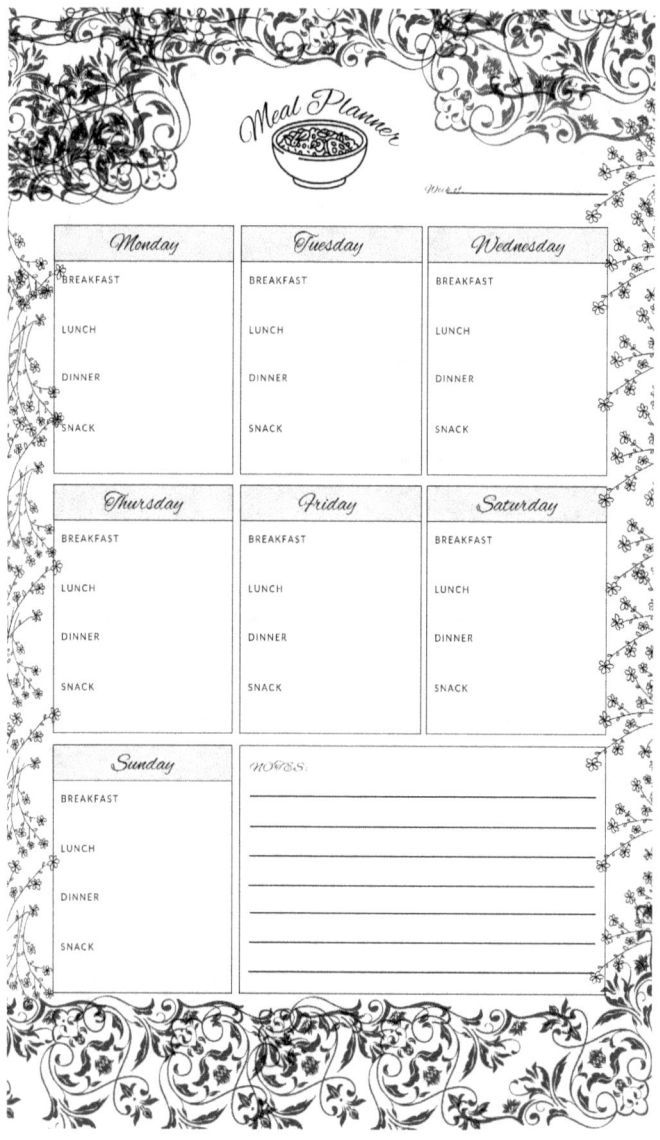

Meal Planner

Week _____

Monday
BREAKFAST

LUNCH

DINNER

SNACK

Tuesday
BREAKFAST

LUNCH

DINNER

SNACK

Wednesday
BREAKFAST

LUNCH

DINNER

SNACK

Thursday
BREAKFAST

LUNCH

DINNER

SNACK

Friday
BREAKFAST

LUNCH

DINNER

SNACK

Saturday
BREAKFAST

LUNCH

DINNER

SNACK

Sunday
BREAKFAST

LUNCH

DINNER

SNACK

NOTES:

_____
_____
_____
_____
_____
_____

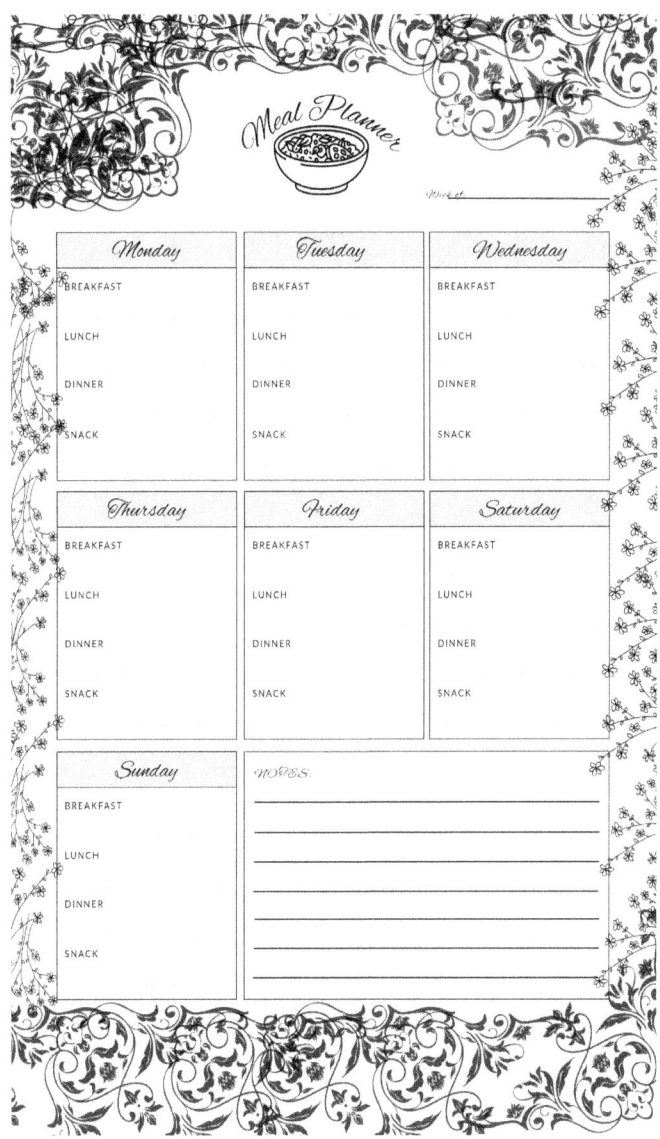

Meal Planner

Week of _____

Monday
BREAKFAST

LUNCH

DINNER

SNACK

Tuesday
BREAKFAST

LUNCH

DINNER

SNACK

Wednesday
BREAKFAST

LUNCH

DINNER

SNACK

Thursday
BREAKFAST

LUNCH

DINNER

SNACK

Friday
BREAKFAST

LUNCH

DINNER

SNACK

Saturday
BREAKFAST

LUNCH

DINNER

SNACK

Sunday
BREAKFAST

LUNCH

DINNER

SNACK

NOTES:

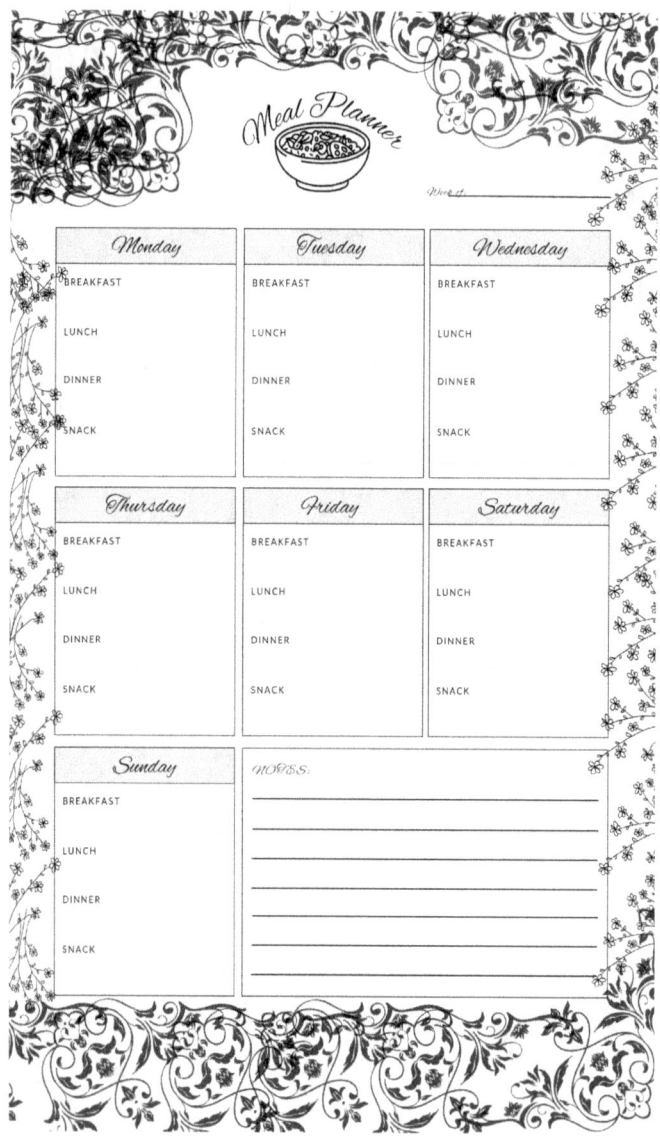

Meal Planner

Week of: _____

Monday
BREAKFAST

LUNCH

DINNER

SNACK

Tuesday
BREAKFAST

LUNCH

DINNER

SNACK

Wednesday
BREAKFAST

LUNCH

DINNER

SNACK

Thursday
BREAKFAST

LUNCH

DINNER

SNACK

Friday
BREAKFAST

LUNCH

DINNER

SNACK

Saturday
BREAKFAST

LUNCH

DINNER

SNACK

Sunday
BREAKFAST

LUNCH

DINNER

SNACK

NOTES:
_____
_____
_____
_____
_____
_____

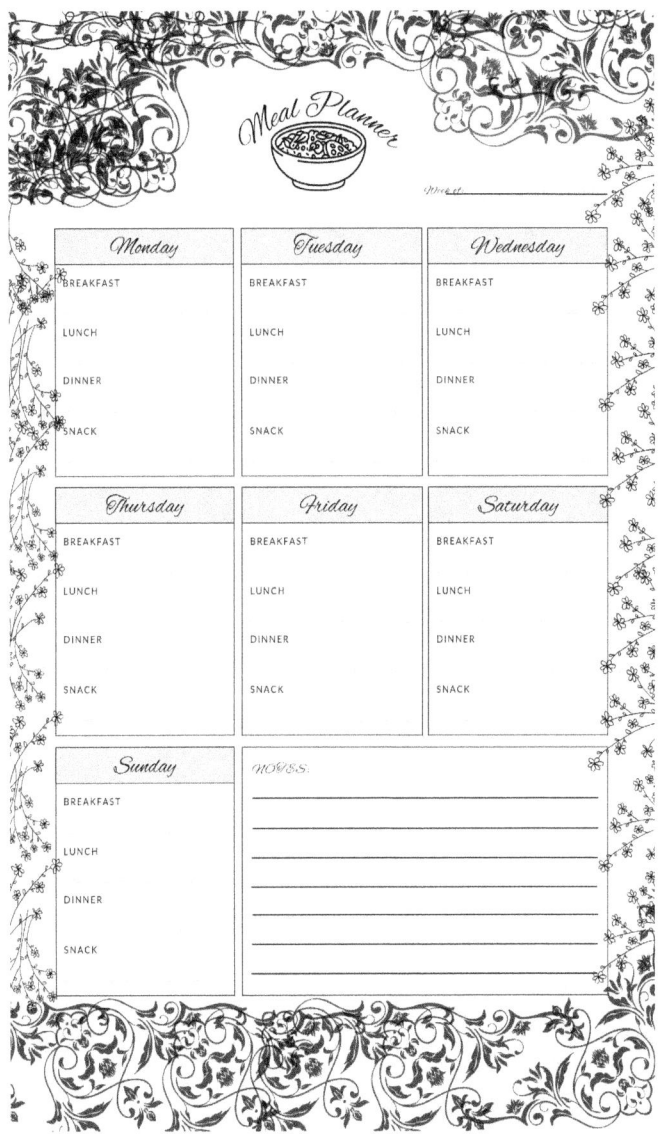

Meal Planner

Week: _____

Monday
BREAKFAST

LUNCH

DINNER

SNACK

Tuesday
BREAKFAST

LUNCH

DINNER

SNACK

Wednesday
BREAKFAST

LUNCH

DINNER

SNACK

Thursday
BREAKFAST

LUNCH

DINNER

SNACK

Friday
BREAKFAST

LUNCH

DINNER

SNACK

Saturday
BREAKFAST

LUNCH

DINNER

SNACK

Sunday
BREAKFAST

LUNCH

DINNER

SNACK

NOTES:
_____
_____
_____
_____
_____
_____
_____
_____

124

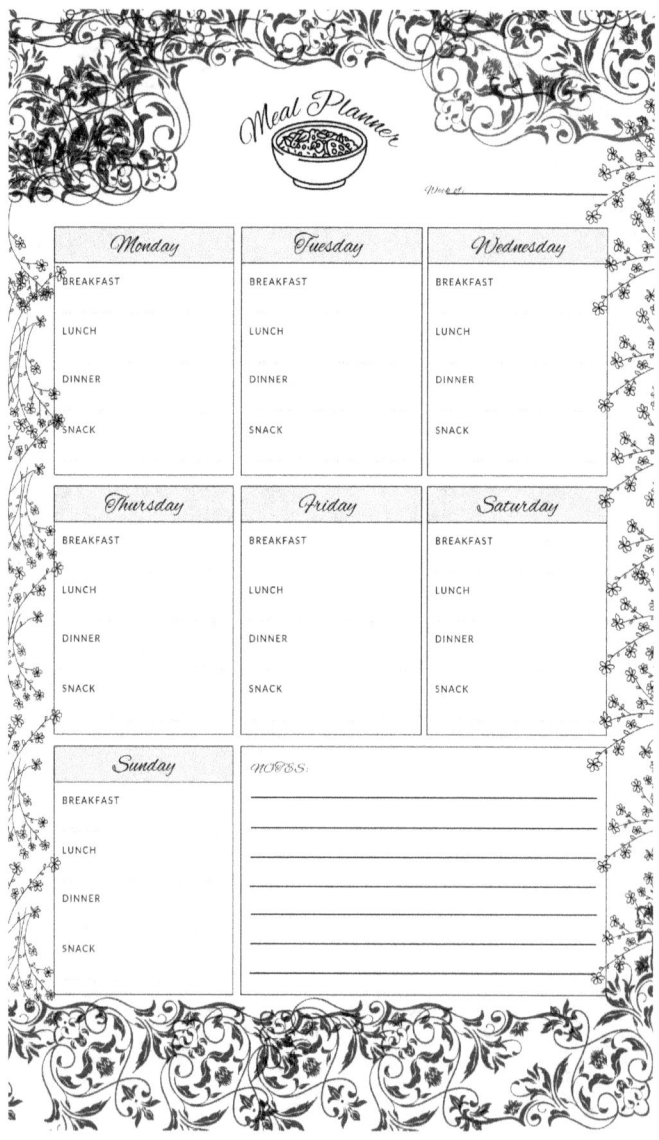

Meal Planner

Week: _____

Monday
BREAKFAST

LUNCH

DINNER

SNACK

Tuesday
BREAKFAST

LUNCH

DINNER

SNACK

Wednesday
BREAKFAST

LUNCH

DINNER

SNACK

Thursday
BREAKFAST

LUNCH

DINNER

SNACK

Friday
BREAKFAST

LUNCH

DINNER

SNACK

Saturday
BREAKFAST

LUNCH

DINNER

SNACK

Sunday
BREAKFAST

LUNCH

DINNER

SNACK

NOTES:
_____
_____
_____
_____
_____
_____
_____

125

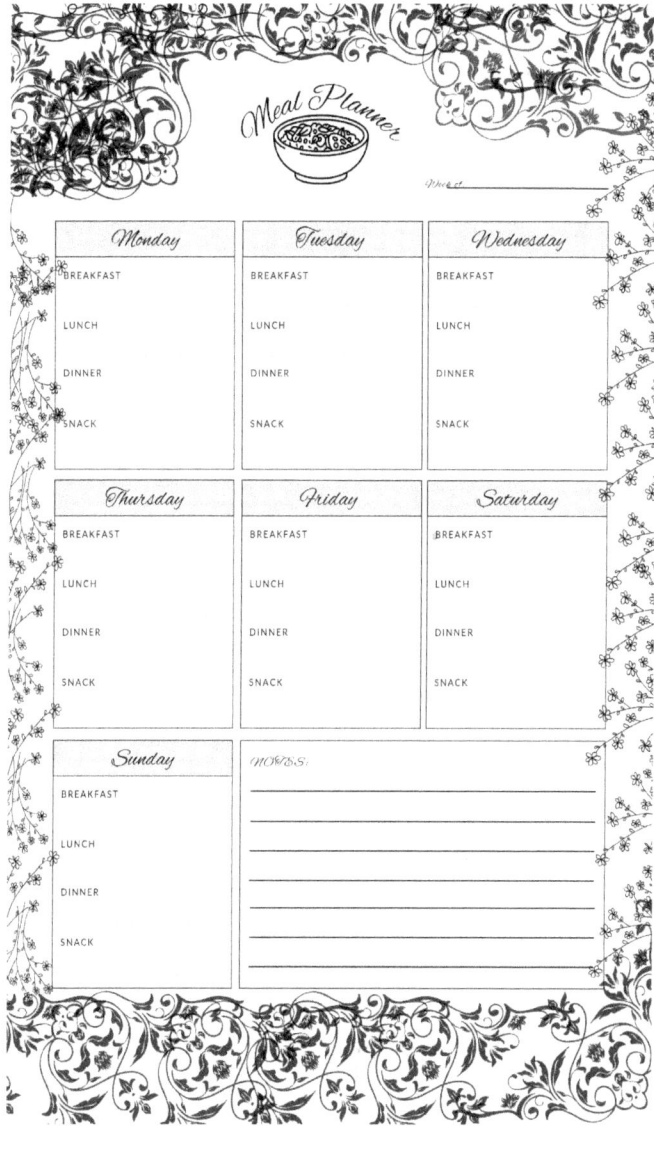

Meal Planner

Week:

Monday
BREAKFAST

LUNCH

DINNER

SNACK

Tuesday
BREAKFAST

LUNCH

DINNER

SNACK

Wednesday
BREAKFAST

LUNCH

DINNER

SNACK

Thursday
BREAKFAST

LUNCH

DINNER

SNACK

Friday
BREAKFAST

LUNCH

DINNER

SNACK

Saturday
BREAKFAST

LUNCH

DINNER

SNACK

Sunday
BREAKFAST

LUNCH

DINNER

SNACK

NOTES:

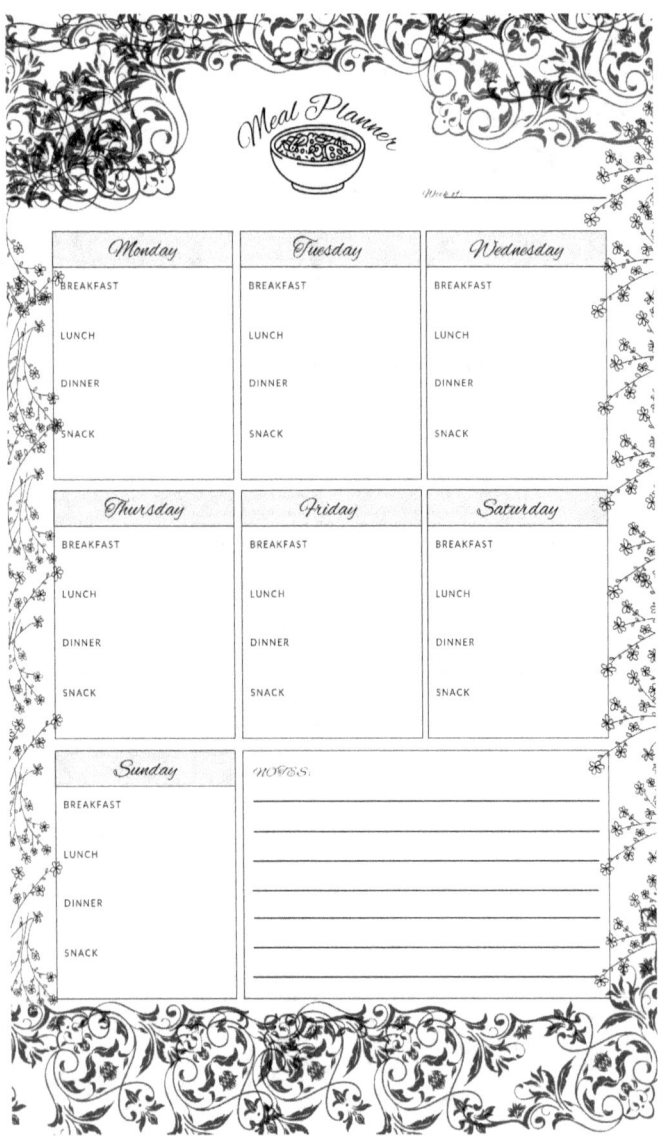

Meal Planner

Week of _____

Monday
BREAKFAST

LUNCH

DINNER

SNACK

Tuesday
BREAKFAST

LUNCH

DINNER

SNACK

Wednesday
BREAKFAST

LUNCH

DINNER

SNACK

Thursday
BREAKFAST

LUNCH

DINNER

SNACK

Friday
BREAKFAST

LUNCH

DINNER

SNACK

Saturday
BREAKFAST

LUNCH

DINNER

SNACK

Sunday
BREAKFAST

LUNCH

DINNER

SNACK

NOTES:
_____
_____
_____
_____
_____
_____
_____

127

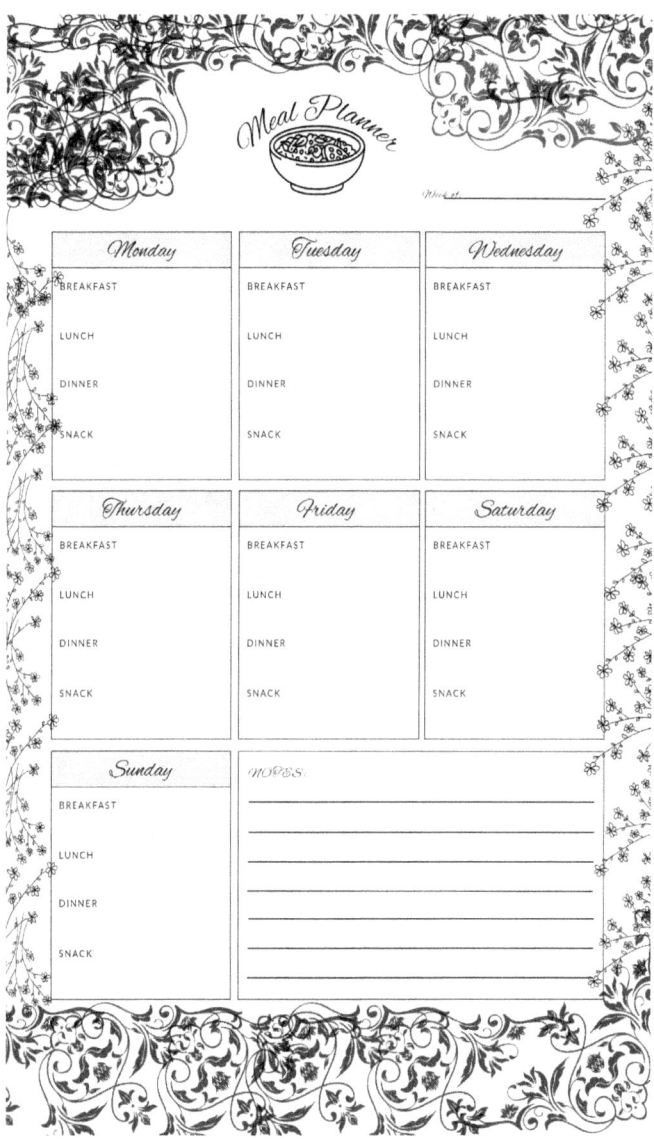

Meal Planner

Week of _____

Monday
BREAKFAST

LUNCH

DINNER

SNACK

Tuesday
BREAKFAST

LUNCH

DINNER

SNACK

Wednesday
BREAKFAST

LUNCH

DINNER

SNACK

Thursday
BREAKFAST

LUNCH

DINNER

SNACK

Friday
BREAKFAST

LUNCH

DINNER

SNACK

Saturday
BREAKFAST

LUNCH

DINNER

SNACK

Sunday
BREAKFAST

LUNCH

DINNER

SNACK

NOTES:

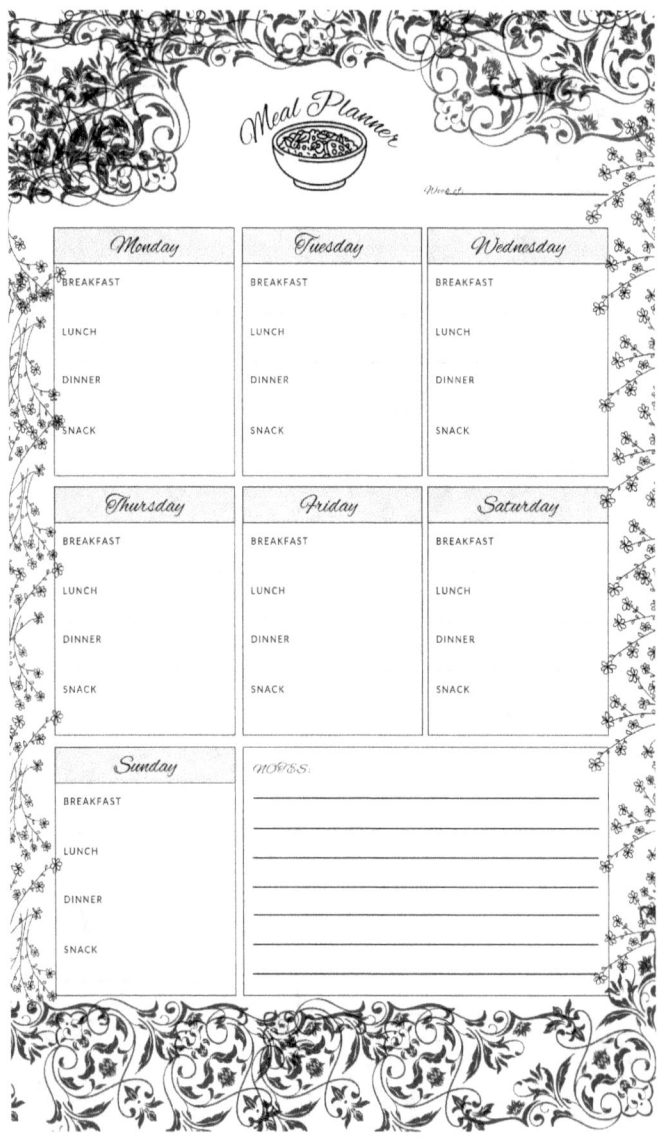

Meal Planner

Week:

Monday
BREAKFAST

LUNCH

DINNER

SNACK

Tuesday
BREAKFAST

LUNCH

DINNER

SNACK

Wednesday
BREAKFAST

LUNCH

DINNER

SNACK

Thursday
BREAKFAST

LUNCH

DINNER

SNACK

Friday
BREAKFAST

LUNCH

DINNER

SNACK

Saturday
BREAKFAST

LUNCH

DINNER

SNACK

Sunday
BREAKFAST

LUNCH

DINNER

SNACK

NOTES:

_____

_____

_____

_____

_____

_____

_____

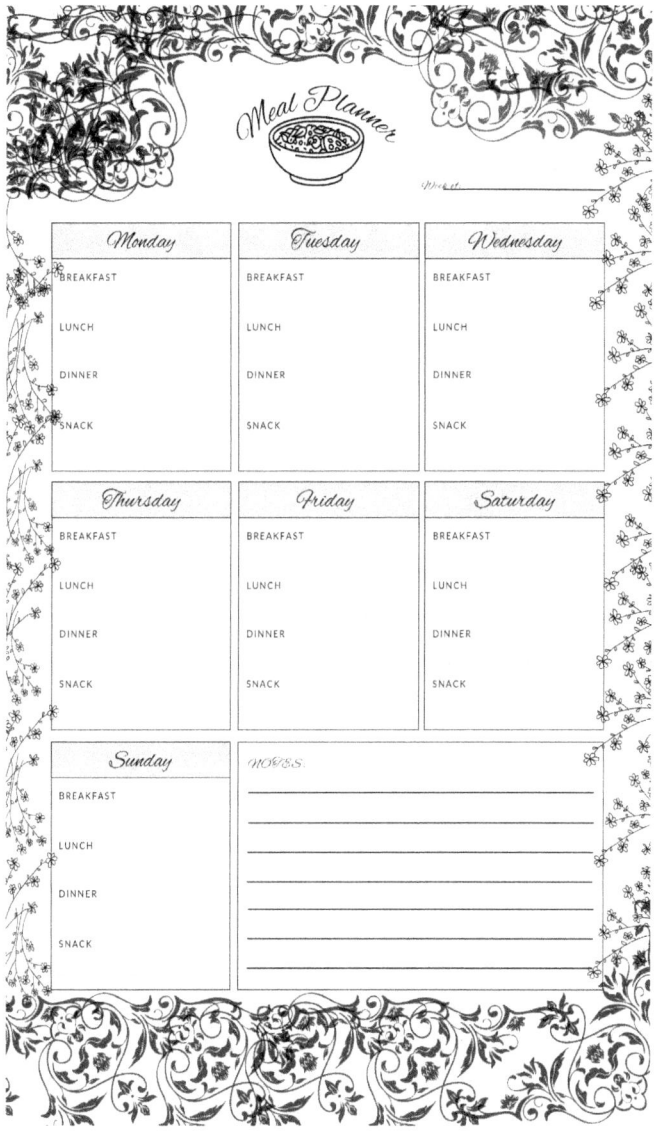

Meal Planner

Week: _____

Monday
BREAKFAST

LUNCH

DINNER

SNACK

Tuesday
BREAKFAST

LUNCH

DINNER

SNACK

Wednesday
BREAKFAST

LUNCH

DINNER

SNACK

Thursday
BREAKFAST

LUNCH

DINNER

SNACK

Friday
BREAKFAST

LUNCH

DINNER

SNACK

Saturday
BREAKFAST

LUNCH

DINNER

SNACK

Sunday
BREAKFAST

LUNCH

DINNER

SNACK

NOTES:
_____
_____
_____
_____
_____
_____
_____

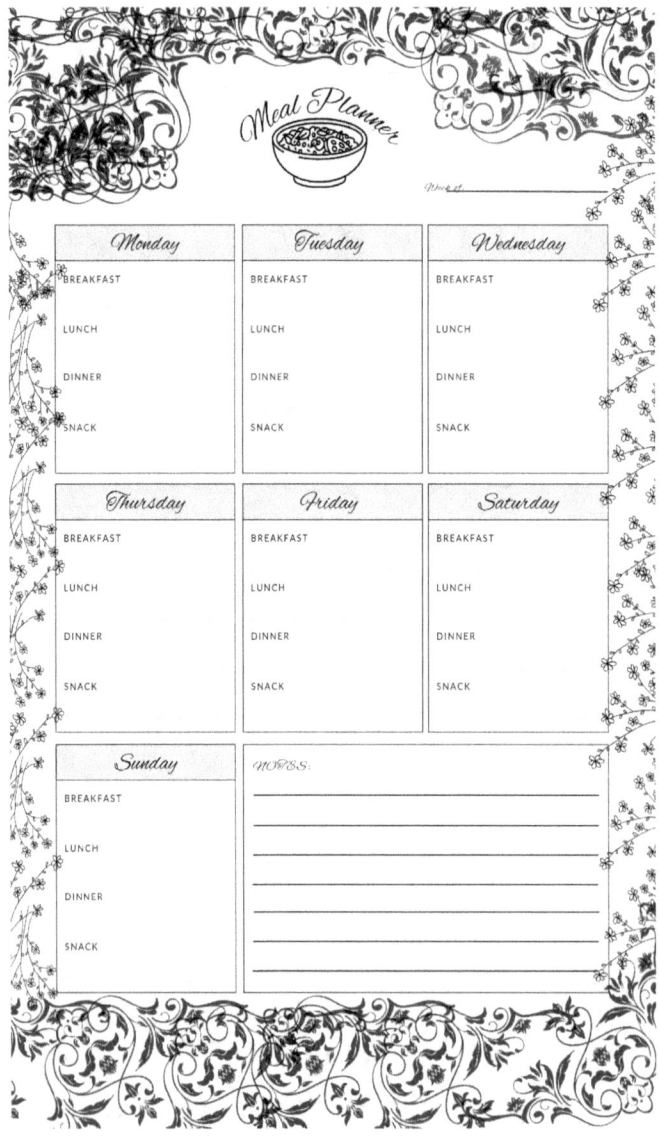

Meal Planner

Week of: _____

Monday
BREAKFAST

LUNCH

DINNER

SNACK

Tuesday
BREAKFAST

LUNCH

DINNER

SNACK

Wednesday
BREAKFAST

LUNCH

DINNER

SNACK

Thursday
BREAKFAST

LUNCH

DINNER

SNACK

Friday
BREAKFAST

LUNCH

DINNER

SNACK

Saturday
BREAKFAST

LUNCH

DINNER

SNACK

Sunday
BREAKFAST

LUNCH

DINNER

SNACK

NOTES:
_____
_____
_____
_____
_____
_____
_____
_____

131